MASSAGE FOR THERAPISTS

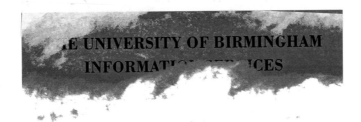

MASSAGE FOR THERAPISTS

Second Edition

Margaret Hollis
MBE, MSc, MCSP, DipTP
Former Principal,
Bradford Hospitals School
of Physiotherapy

Blackwell
Science

19671474

© 1987, 1998 by
Blackwell Science Ltd
Editorial Offices:
Osney Mead, Oxford OX2 0EL
25 John Street, London WC1N 2BL
23 Ainslie Place, Edinburgh EH3 6AJ
350 Main Street, Malden
   MA 02148 5018, USA
54 University Street, Carlton
   Victoria 3053, Australia
10, rue Casimir Delavigne
   75006 Paris, France

Other Editorial Offices:

Blackwell Wissenschafts-Verlag GmbH
Kurfürstendamm 57
10707 Berlin, Germany

Blackwell Science KK
MG Kodenmacho Building
7-10 Kodenmacho Nihombashi
Chuo-ku, Tokyo 104, Japan

First edition published 1987
Reprinted 1988, 1990, 1992, 1993, 1996
Second edition published 1998

Set in Sabon 10 on 13.5 pt
by Best-set Typesetter Ltd., Hong Kong
Printed and bound in Great Britain
at The Alden Press, Oxford

DISTRIBUTORS

Marston Book Services Ltd
PO Box 269
Abingdon
Oxon OX14 4YN
(*Orders:* Tel: 01235 465500
          Fax: 01235 465555)

USA
Blackwell Science, Inc.
Commerce Place
350 Main Street
Malden, MA 02148 5018
(*Orders:* Tel: 800 759 6102
                781 388 8250
          Fax: 781 388 8255)

Canada
Login Brothers Book Company
324 Saulteaux Crescent
Winnipeg, Manitoba R3J 3T2
(*Orders:* Tel: 204 224-4068)

Australia
Blackwell Science Pty Ltd
54 University Street
Carlton, Victoria 3053
(*Orders:* Tel: 03 9347 0300
          Fax: 03 9347 5001)

A catalogue record for this title
is available from the British Library

ISBN 0-632-04788-7

Library of Congress
Cataloging-in-Publication Data

Hollis, Margaret.
    Massage for therapists/Margaret Hollis. – 2nd
    ed.
        p.   cm.
    Includes bibliographical references and index.
    ISBN 0-632-04788-7
    1. Massage therapy.   I. Title.
RM721.H58   1998
615.8′22 – dc21   98-15039
                                          CIP

For further information on
Blackwell Science, visit our website:
www.blackwell-science.com

CONTENTS

PREFACE TO
SECOND EDITION

I have been fortunate for this edition to enlist the services of colleagues. Elizabeth Jones has written a chapter on Aromatherapy and Joan M. Watt has written a chapter on Massage in Sport and both enhance the book. I am very grateful for their contributions.

We had just embarked on the revision when Alison Walker, who was to revise Chapter 3, on effects, sadly died. Using some of Alison's research, Janice M. Warriner has taken over and revised this chapter for me and I am very grateful for her efforts which also enhance the book.

I did not need to revise the chapters on techniques as I had originally described what I taught and what I in turn had learnt from my teachers. There are no references for this section as it is 'out of my head'. I have added a chapter on massage to the abdomen which my colleagues are eager to have as it is increasingly used in place of laxatives for constipation, especially in the physically and mentally handicapped. There has been some revision of the other treatment sections.

Peter Harrison undertook the new photography, Sheila Middlemiss came to model for us and Janice Eccles has again typed the manuscript. I am grateful to all of them for their help.

Margaret Hollis

NOTE TO THE READER

In this book Part I is intended for the student of massage who will I hope spend many hours practising on a model – hopefully a fellow student able to be aware of the 'feel' of the manipulations and thus able to comment constructively to the practitioner. Part II is about treatments for particular states or conditions. While these should be practised first on a model they will be used on patients or on sportsmen and sportswomen for specific effects. Thus in the early chapters I have referred to the recipient as the model and later on as the patient. Where techniques are practised on a model for use on a patient I have used both terms. I have hesitated to use the word 'client' which may be modern usage but can have unfortunate connotations in some circumstances! I have made the assumption that some knowledge of anatomy has already been achieved by readers.

Part I

THE MANIPULATIONS AND THEIR EFFECTS

Chapter 1
PREPARATION FOR MASSAGE

Massage is referred to by some people as an art, perhaps because its practice involves co-ordination of a high order and the use of great skill to achieve the integrated body movements which allow the application of the appropriate manipulations at the correct depth and speed to achieve maximum effect. To this end the potential practitioner must practise each manipulation with great awareness of their own contact with the subject, whether model or patient, so that any discomfort is immediately noticed and the cause detected. Uncomfortable massage is usually born of failure of co-ordinated performance by the practitioner. Minor adjustment of foot position and trunk posture will change the relationship of the practitioner to the support and the subject; and the totality of hand contact and the angle of contact will be altered by the posture of the trunk and arms. Finally, weight transference from the practitioner's feet to the subject will control depth. Rhythm must then be considered, as uneven movement of any one of the practitioner's body components will cause uneven contact, jerky movements of the whole line of work and angular patterns which will cause uneven compression or dragging by some part of the working hand.

Thus when starting to perform and practise massage check that you can:

- Reach all parts
- Stand in walk or lunge standing to do so

- Change position from that shown in Fig. 1.1 to that shown in Fig. 1.2 without impedance or hesitation

Self preparation

The practitioner should start preparation of himself or herself long before contact with the model/patient. Attention to personal appearance, hygiene and manicure are all important. As close contact will inevitably occur, the practitioner should wear protective clothing which is easily laundered and which allows freedom of movement while maintaining decency. Long

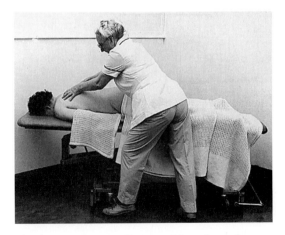

Fig. 1.1 Lunge standing reaching along the length of the body.

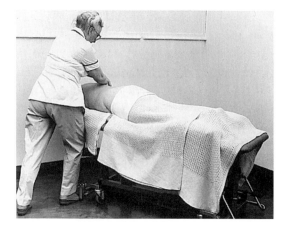

Fig. 1.2 Walk standing reaching across the body.

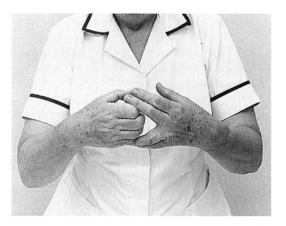

Fig. 1.3 Exercise to increase hand span.

hair must be restrained so that it cannot come into contact with the subject and, equally, necklaces or other jewellery which can dangle should be discarded as should a wristwatch. Rings should be removed as they can cause discomfort to the practitioner when performing some manipulations and to the model/patient during most manipulations. Thin wedding rings may be the exception to this rule – provided they do not cause discomfort to anyone. Well cared for hands which are smooth, with short, clean nails are essential.

Cleanliness is important so wash your hands before and after each treatment. Cultivate warm hands by always using warm water for washing and it also helps to keep your hands covered when outside in the cold.

The range of movements of all the joints of your forearm and hands should be full. If you have stiff hands, do a series of stretching exercises aimed at increasing your range of movement. The most important large range movements are:

- Full abduction/extension of the thumb to give a wide grasp – an octave span

- Full flexion and extension of the wrists or at least 80° of each movement
- Full pronation and supination of the radio-ulnar joints.

Hand exercises

To obtain these ranges of movement the following exercises should be practised. Before each exercise check your shoulder relaxation:

(1) Touch the finger tips of one hand with the finger tips of the other and press so that your thumbs and little fingers are separated widely.
(2) Push the fist of one hand between two adjacent fingers of the other hand so that they are separated into wider abduction. Keep your fingers in the same plane. Repeat for each space (Fig. 1.3).
(3) Place your hands together as in prayer and with your thumbs resting on your chest push your wrists downwards to extend them without separating the heels of your hands.
(4) Reverse your hands, placing the backs together and push your elbows downwards thus flexing your wrists.
(5) Place your hands in the prayer position and, keeping them together, turn them

down and up. Try to touch your abdomen and chest alternately at each rotation. When you can hold the full extension with your hands just very slightly separated practise the rotation of your two hands, not touching, but simultaneously. Next move your two hands alternately so that they pass one another at mid-point (Fig. 1.4). Observe that the finger tips of each hand will now strike your abdomen at precisely the same point.

Relaxation

Relaxation of your hands is very important so that you always use your hands in full contact with your model/patient, and moulded to the shape of the body you are touching, with awareness of the tissues and of their state.

Relaxed hand contact is one in which the hand conforms to the contour of the part. The natural rest position of the human hand is with the fingers and thumb a little apart and very slightly flexed at each joint and it can easily be adjusted to allow contact with any size of body part. This is the contact which is used in many massage manipulations.

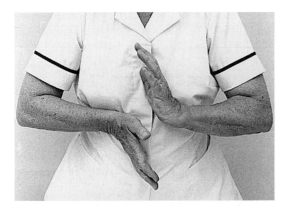

Fig. 1.4 The ultimate ability is to maintain wrist extension with a relaxed hand and perform full range pronation and supination with alternate hands.

In addition you will need to be able to relax your whole arm to perform some manipulations. You should practise a method of relaxation yourself prior to learning massage. A good method is reciprocal relaxation as you will then become more aware of the position of all your joints and be capable of local relaxation of any body part as needed. Briefly, reciprocal relaxation involves working the opposite muscles to those you wish to relax, then stopping the action and appreciating the new, relaxed position of that body part (Hollis 1993).

Co-ordinated and integrated movement of your body is essential for the comfortable and prolonged performance of massage manipulations without fatigue and physical stress on the practitioner.

You should stand in walk standing and practise transferring your weight forwards and backwards while maintaining your arms stretched away from you:

- Across the couch as in Fig. 1.2
- Along the couch as in Fig. 1.1

These movements, along the length of the model/patient and across the model/patient, are key movements in massage. The former allows you to practise long, reaching actions with variable weight from your hands on to the length of the body structures; the latter allows you to practise short, reaching actions with variable weight from your hands across the length of the body structures.

The environment

The treatment area should be well heated and well ventilated but not draughty. The padded treatment couch may be covered with fresh linen.

Linen you may need

- An underblanket and a covering cotton sheet
- Large and small washable blankets and/or sheets
- Standard size pillows and pillow covers
- Small or half size pillows and pillow covers

Treatment couch

An adjustable height couch is most useful, of the type that has an elevating mechanism at each end and a removable section to accommodate the nose when the model/patient is in prone lying. The couch should be covered with an underblanket if it is made of 'cold' material, with a cotton sheet on top. You may find it more manageable to anchor these covers with a series of flat straps, checking that the fastenings are under the couch and not in contact with the model/patient.

Contact materials

Powder

- Talcum powder is the commonest contact medium. It should be non-perfumed if possible, or a baby powder may be selected.
- Corn Starch BP, which is sterilisable, is a heavy powder which absorbs sweat very readily and should be used in the presence of profound sweating by either the model/patient or the practitioner.

Oils

- Pure lanolin – which has a 'drag' effect on skin due to its thick and heavy texture is used to obtain a slight pull on the skin. Lanolin cream which is a water based cream is used when less 'drag' is required.

- Liquid oils – the most commonly used liquid oil is probably olive oil, and liquid paraffin may also be used to provide a 'gliding' effect and to lubricate the skin. The disadvantage of such oils is that they become rancid and, if left in contact with the skin, can smell offensive. Other oils are dealt with in Chapter 10.

Water-based lubricants

The water-based lubricant most commonly used is ung. eucerin. This light cream is used to give moderate lubrication and, as it absorbs rapidly, is mainly of value as an introduction to deeper work.

The thinner oils used in massage tend to reduce the depth at which the practitioner can work as the hands glide on the lubricated skin and slide away from the part being treated, instead of working with depth. Thicker oils do not cause this problem. Note also that the smaller the manipulations you perform when using oils, the more likely you are to obtain greater depth.

Soap and water

Soap and hot water, with or without the addition of oil, is used for scaly skins which may be caused by prolonged immobilisation in a cast or by use of some medications which promote and increase skin healing and at the same time cause the skin to become dry and scaly.

Preparation of the patient/model

Ask the patient/model to undress so that the part to be treated is adequately uncovered. Remember that some manipulations, to be effective, must extend to the lymph glands lying in proximal spaces. Thus:

For treatment of the upper limb, unclothe from the neck to finger tips and especially remove all straps.

For treatment of the lower limb, unclothe from the groin to the toe – remove trousers, do not pull them up.

For treatment of the back, unclothe from the head to the buttocks. Pants/briefs can remain on, but must be pulled down to leave the area above the gluteal cleft exposed.

For treatment of the neck, unclothe from the head to the level of the lowest point of origin of trapezius, i.e. 12th thoracic vertebra.

For treatment of the face, unclothe from the hairline to just below the clavicle.

Ensure the patient/model is kept warm by the use of coverings, e.g. if he or she is sitting, wrap him or her in a blanket leaving the arm part to be treated free (Fig. 2.3). If the patient/model is to lie down cover him or her immediately, having first placed pillows in position as needed. The patient in lying may need:

• One or two head pillows
• A pillow under the knees (Fig. 2.16)

The patient in prone lying may need:

• Two head pillows crossing one another to create an inverted and open triangle so that his or her nose rests below the crossing
• A pillow under the abdomen to raise and thus flatten the lumbar spine (Fig. 6.1)
• A pillow under the ankles to flex the knees slightly

More pillows will be needed for special positions and these are dealt with in the treatments section.

If you use one large cover initially ensure that smaller covers are on hand so that you can split them to keep the patient/model covered and warm.

Small sheets are very useful for placing in direct contact with the patient/model and to protect the blankets. Sheets are more easily washed and less likely to retain any powder you may use.

Palpation and developing sensory awareness (Hollis & Yung 1985)

Palpation is a skill that is acquired by practice. It requires that your hands should be relaxed, in firm comfortable contact, and aware of what is under them. The term 'thinking hands' implies that your mind is envisaging the structures that your hands are feeling and is alert both to identify the structure and become aware of variations from normal in the state of the structure.

To learn how to palpate, practise the following procedures. Place your whole hand on a series of varying size, rounded structures in turn, starting with large ones that require an almost flat hand, for example:

• A cushion or part-filled hot water bottle
• A smaller bottle or rolling pin
• A broomstick handle

Increase your pressure on the object to grasp firmly with your whole hand, modifying your hand posture so that every part of the palmar surface is in contact simultaneously. Then release your pressure very slowly until you are only just grasping – think hard about the quality of this pressure. Next, release your pressure so that the object could start to slip. Think about and appreciate this pressure, as such pressure is likely to tickle the patient.

Following this, enlist the help of a colleague and repeat the procedure, applying in turn very firm, firm and very light contact on the back, the thigh, the calf, the arm, the forearm and the foot. Appreciate what pressure/contact you need to be able to touch and not hurt, and to touch and not tickle.

Again use a colleague and decide to palpate for specific anatomical features. Place more of your hand than you need in contact with the area to be examined, lift your palm a little to reduce the contact, so that only the finger pads are touching firmly enough. Your fingers should be straight so that your nails are unlikely to be in contact. Do not lose contact, but, if you do, refrain from re-establishing it by putting only your finger tips on again. To do so will cause you either to poke and hurt or to tickle by touching again too lightly. Remember that too hard a pressure will feel like a drill digging in (Fig. 1.5) and too light a pressure will feel like a butterfly coming to rest (Fig. 1.6). In neither case will you feel or find anything.

Now slide your fingers towards the structure to be palpated and in doing so ensure that your pressure is such that you neither drag the skin nor skid over it. Mentally count off the anatomical landmarks and apply the check tests that you have learned for identifying that structure, for example:

(1) Arteries can be felt to pulsate
(2) Pressure on veins occludes them so that they appear most full distally
(3) Tendons have muscle tissue attached that can contract and act
(4) Ligamentous structures can be made to appear or disappear in different positions of joints

Examination of the part

Before performing massage on either a model on whom you will practise or a patient whom

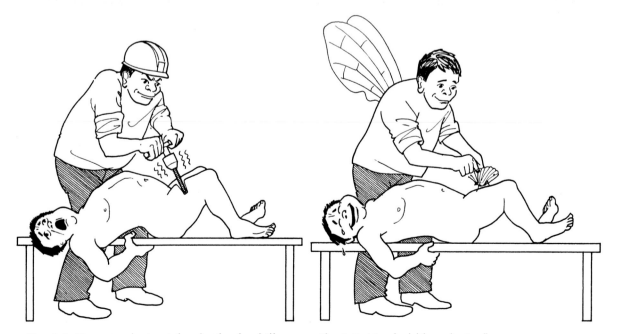

Fig. 1.5 Do not palpate at the depth of a drill.   **Fig. 1.6** Nor feel like a butterfly.

you will treat you should examine the part on which you are going to work. In the case of a patient you will, of course, have carried out a complete examination and assessment so that you are aware of the problems which the patient presents.

Whether working on a model or a patient, having arranged him or her as described above, you should now examine the part you intend to massage.

Look at the skin state for dryness, oiliness, wetness, hairiness and completeness – thus you observe bruises, abrasions and lacerations. Look also at the state of subcutaneous tissues - is the skin emaciated or well padded and if the former, is it taut? Is there any oedema or excess reddening?

Feel – Run your hand down the length of the part on every aspect. **Think** as you do so and be aware not only of the temperature of each area, the degree of muscle tension and joint posture but of any flinching as painful or ticklish areas are touched. Make mental notes so that problem areas can be approached with caution.

Ticklish subjects

People who are ticklish can be massaged without discomfort to them provided you observe the rules of always putting your hands in very firm contact as you start work and never lifting your hands off by 'trickling', i.e. by lifting your palms off first, then each phalanx, until only your finger tips are in contact.

You should also never move one hand component, especially fingers, in relation to one another once you have placed your hands in contact.

Light work tickles, so always perform the manipulations at the maximum depth tolerable by the model/patient and to produce the required result.

References

Hollis, M. (1993) *Practical Exercise Therapy*, 3rd edn, pp. 33–4. Blackwell Science Ltd, Oxford.

Hollis, M. & Yung, P. (1985) *Patient Examination and Assessment for Therapists*, pp. 12–15. Blackwell Science Ltd, Oxford.

Chapter 2
THE MASSAGE MANIPULATIONS

The manipulations described in this chapter are:

- The effleurage/stroking manipulations
- The petrissage manipulations
- The friction manipulations
- The percussive (tapôtement) manipulations

The effleurage/stroking manipulations

The word 'effleurage' means to stroke, and the manipulations in this group may be divided into:

(1) Those in which the intention is primarily to assist venous and lymphatic drainage and in which the direction of the work is from distal to proximal – usually called effleurage.

(2) Those in which the intention is primarily to obtain a sensory reaction either sedative or stimulative and in which direction is not important but is often from proximal to distal – usually called stroking.

In this book the words effleurage and stroking will apply to the above respective descriptions.

Effleurage

Effleurage is a unidirectional manipulation in which the operator's hand passes from distal to proximal with a depth compatible with the state of the tissues and the desired effect. Thus, the manipulation may start at one end and proceed to the proximal space, draining the part to be treated, e.g. finger tips to axilla, toes to groin, buttocks to axilla, neck to supraclavicular glands. The depth should be such as to push fluid onwards in the superficial vessels. This may be observed especially in the veins of the forearm. The manipulation is performed with the whole hand softly curved and relaxed to fit the part, or with any part of the hand which fits the part. Both hands may be used together (Fig. 2.1) on opposite aspects of a part, or may follow one another (Fig. 2.2). Each hand may be used singly while the opposite hand supports the part in an appropriate position (Fig. 2.3). As the manipulation proceeds over the part, the hand(s) must change shape to maintain perfect contact.

The stance of the operator is very important as these manipulations often proceed over a considerable length of the body, and it must be possible for the operator to transfer body weight to and fro. Walk standing (Fig. 1.2) is the usual stance adopted, with the weight being transferred from the rear to the forward foot accompanied, if need be, by either or both

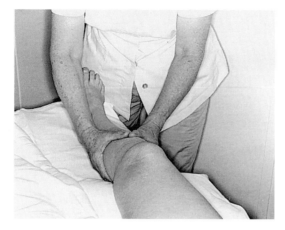

Fig. 2.1 Effleurage using both hands together on opposite aspects.

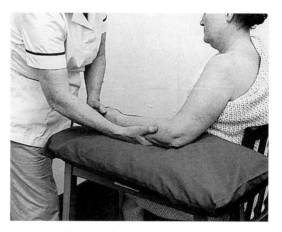

Fig. 2.3 Effleurage using one hand while the other hand supports.

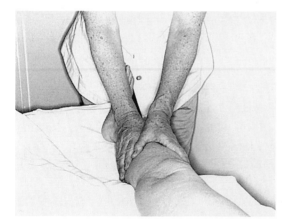

Fig. 2.2 Effleurage using both hands together following one another.

lifting of the heel of the rear foot and flexion and extension of the knees and hips (Fig. 1.1). The arms will initially be flexed and become more extended, especially at the elbows as the 'reach' is made. Integration of the arm and body movements must be obtained to ensure a smooth movement of the hand along the part; this is achieved if the arms stretch first followed by the body weight transfer. At the end of every

line of effleurage there should be a small increase in depth (often called overpressure) and a slight pause (in the space) before the hand is lifted off with minimum flourish and returned to the distal part to start the next line of work. Some people advocate stroking the hand back to the start. The disadvantage of this method can be either a tickling effect if the return stroke is too light or a feeling of downdrag if the return stroke is too deep.

When the whole hand is used for effleurage, it does not maintain equal contact over its whole surface and should be placed obliquely on the skin so that the leading edge is the 'C' formed by the thumb to forefinger cleft. This edge is formed by the lateral border of the forefinger and the medial border of the thumb linked by the adjacent web; however, the main pressure is exerted by the 'C' formed by the lateral border of the thumb, the thenar eminence, the hypothenar eminence and the little finger. The pressure is graded from the index to little fingers and adjacent parts of the palm so that the hand operates in the manner of a ski.

If the pressure is exerted by the leading edge, it can be uncomfortable or jerky, or can cause sticking. Lack of control of the modulation of the pressure as the hand proceeds up the part is more usually caused by:

either standing too near the finish of the stroke
  (step back to cure this)
or by failing to synchronise the arm movements
  with the weight transfer (see page 11).

Stroking

Stroking is a unidirectional manipulation in which the operator's hand passes, usually, from proximal to distal down the length of the tissues at a depth and speed compatible with the required effect, but direction of the stroke may be varied to give greater comfort.

The stroke should start with firm contact (try not to trickle your fingers on) and finish with a smooth lift off of your hands. The hands may be positioned obliquely or so that the heel travels first, but can adjust its position down the length of the part so that comfortable contact is maintained.

The slower strokes are more sedative. Try a speed of one stroke per five seconds. The faster strokes are more stimulating. Try a speed of four strokes every five seconds, i.e. four times faster.

Obviously greater depth can be achieved at the slower rate, but the need for sedative effects may limit your depth when pain and muscle spasm prevent firmer contact. If this is so, the depth is increased as relaxation occurs and pain diminishes but the tempo should still be maintained. The faster stroking is often used to complete a more stimulating massage.

The whole area under treatment should be covered by a sequence of strokes. Stroking may be performed using:

(1) One hand – usually on a narrow area
(2) Two hands simultaneously – one each side on a broad area – be careful not to pull on the part (Fig. 1.1)
(3) Right and left hands following one another on a narrow area
(4) Thumb(s) or finger(s) on confined areas one-handed, two-handed or alternately
(5) A technique called 'thousand hands' in which one hand performs a short stroke, the second hand does the same overlapping the first, and the hands pass over one another to gain contact as the manipulation proceeds down the length of the part under treatment.

The petrissage manipulation

Petrissage manipulations are those in which the soft tissues (mainly muscles) are compressed either against underlying bone or against themselves. They are divided into:

- **Kneading manipulations** – when the tissues are compressed against the underlying structures
- **Picking up manipulations** – when the tissues are compressed then lifted and squeezed
- **Wringing manipulations** – when the tissues are lifted and squeezed by alternating hand pressure
- **Rolling manipulations** – when the tissues are lifted and rolled between the fingers and thumbs as in skin rolling or muscle rolling
- **Shaking manipulations** – when the tissues are lifted and shaken from side to side

Kneading

Kneading is a circular manipulation performed so that the skin and subcutaneous tissues are moved in a circular manner on the underlying structures. The manipulation may be performed with the palmar aspect of the whole hand, with the palm only, with all the fingers, or with the pads or tips of the thumb or of the fingers. Whatever the area used, a circle is described by the part of your hand in contact, with pressure on the upward part of the circle but only for a small segment. The actual range or number of degrees for which pressure is exerted varies with the part treated.

On flat areas, e.g. the back, the pressure with the right hand is from 8 o'clock to 11 o'clock with that hand circling clockwise. The left hand circles counter clockwise and exerts pressure from 4 o'clock to 1 o'clock (Fig. 2.4). On the limbs, the pressure is exerted from 6 o'clock to 9 o'clock with the right hand and from 6 o'clock to 3 o'clock with the left hand. On the non-pressure phase of the circle the hand maintains contact but glides on to the next area of skin a small enough distance to allow the next circle to cover at least half the previous area. The right hand moving clockwise will slide downwards from 4 o'clock, while the left hand will glide downwards from 8 o'clock (Fig. 2.4). Great care must be taken to transmit the required pressure to get the necessary depth through the whole hand and not just the heel of the hand. This is effected by correct foot position and body position giving a correct relationship to the part under treatment, plus integrated flexion of hips, shoulders and elbows to transfer and use body weight. In performing all kneading manipulations use walk standing so that your body weight can move easily from one foot to the other.

Kneading may be performed with:

(1) The whole hand – whole hand kneading (Fig. 2.5)
(2) The palm only – palmar kneading (Fig. 2.6)

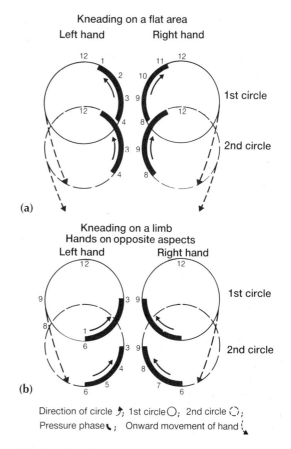

Fig. 2.4 Kneading: the right hand works clockwise and the left hand counterclockwise. Pressure is exerted for the shaded part of the circle only: (a) on a flat area (the back); (b) on a round area (the limbs). The hands move on at the down-pointing arrows.

(3) The fingers only:
   (a) flat finger kneading (Fig. 2.7)
   (b) finger pad kneading (Fig. 2.8)
   (c) finger tip kneading (Fig. 2.9)
(4) The thumb:
   (a) thumb pad kneading (Fig. 2.10)
   (b) thumb tip kneading (Fig. 2.11)
(5) Both hands when one is superimposed on the other – superimposed (reinforced) kneading (Fig. 2.12)
(6) Elbow kneading (Fig. 2.13)
(7) Heel of hand kneading (Fig. 2.14)

In the case of the first four options, the manipulation may be performed:

- Single-handed (Fig. 2.15)
- double-handed – alternately (Fig. 2.5) or simultaneously (Fig. 2.11)

The choice is dictated to some extent by the size of the part under treatment and by the state of the tissues. For example, superimposed kneading has considerable depth and is used on the back and gluteal regions, while thumb and finger tip kneading is used on narrow muscle groups such as the interossei or peronei. But subjects with very mobile skins may not be suitable for simultaneous double-handed kneading as it is too easy to perform a large range manipulation and cause the subject to slide up and down on the bed. This is especially so when working on the back with the subject in prone lying.

Performance

Stand in walk standing.

(1) Whole hand kneading

Place your hand obliquely to the long axis of the part and maintain full contact using all of the palmar surface to perform the manipulation (Fig. 2.5).

(2) Palmar kneading

Use only the palm of your hand and allow your fingers and thumb to relax off-contact with the subject. Great depth can be gained using the palm so take care not to dig in with the bony prominences of the carpus (Fig. 2.6).

(3)(a) Flat finger kneading

This is performed with the palmar surfaces of the second to fifth digits while the palm and thumb remain off-contact. It is often used to

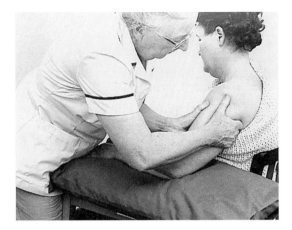

Fig. 2.5 Kneading: using the whole palmar aspect of the hand.

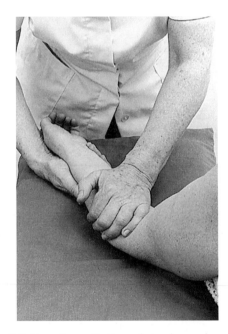

Fig. 2.6 Kneading with the palm only – palmar kneading.

work on less muscular or poorly padded areas (Fig. 2.7).

(3)(b) Finger pad kneading

This is performed with the finger pads either individually, when index or middle fingers are

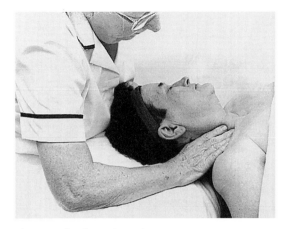

Fig. 2.7 Flat finger kneading.

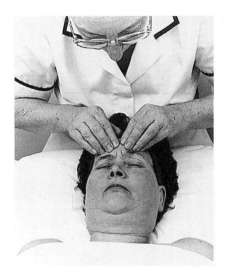

Fig. 2.8 Finger pad kneading.

more commonly used, or with several finger pads together to provide a linear contact (Fig. 2.8). The little finger may be too short on most people so the index, middle and ring fingers are bent sufficiently to allow the pads to create a contact line. These manipulations are often used round joints and along the line of ligaments and in treating scars.

(3)(c) *Finger tip kneading*

This is performed in the same way as finger pad kneading but using only the tip of the pad, taking care to keep your nails off-contact (Fig. 2.9). Narrow, linear areas are dealt with using several finger tips, and one finger tip should be used on small structures or to work on painful areas when the patient will tolerate only very small contact and no movement of the part.

(4)(a) *Thumb kneading*

This is performed with the thumb pads. The size of the area to be treated dictates the amount of the pad which is in contact with the subject's skin. On the larger areas, such as the forearm, back and leg, the whole pad is used (Fig. 2.10). The manipulation is usually per-

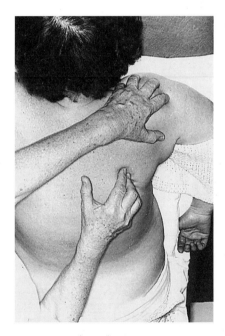

Fig. 2.9 Finger tip kneading.

formed by resting your fingers on the opposite side of the limbs or more laterally on the back, but when working on the face, or in the presence of any contra-indications, the fingers

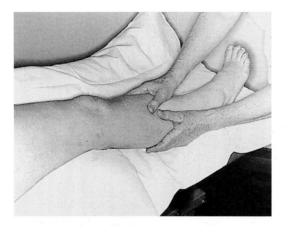

Fig. 2.10 Thumb pad kneading.

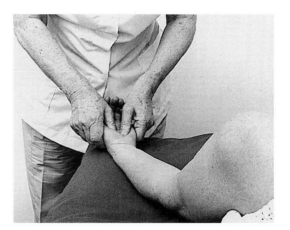

Fig. 2.11 Thumb tip kneading.

should not rest on the subject. The skin and subcutaneous tissues should be moved on the underlying tissues so as to produce a wrinkle on the outer sides of the working thumb (Fig. 2.10). Mobile, well-padded skin allows a greater range circle to be performed.

Note also the position of the working and resting thumbs. Both lie at an angle to the long axis of the limb, the resting thumb in position ready to start the next circle, while the working thumb maintains the same angle but describes a circle. In other words, the thumb angles to the limb or part only change to accommodate the size of the part and the thumb should never slide into adduction.

The working thumb will almost invariably have to pass the resting thumb and should do so by slipping past its tip in contact. If the thumb is lifted to move on, then a 'cat walking' effect is produced, the length of the thumb contact is lost and the pressure of the manipulation will be more likely to be too deep, uneven and less effective.

(4)(b)   *Thumb tip kneading* (Fig. 2.11)

This is performed more frequently with the side of the thumb tip and is useful when the part to

be treated has a long, narrow shape – as the interosseus spaces. Your fingers act as counter supports on the opposite aspect of the part and your thumb should lie in adduction so that your lateral thumb tip is in contact without involving your nail (Fig. 5.10).

(5)   *Superimposed (re-inforced) kneading*

This type of kneading can be very deep and is usually performed when greater depth is required. The contact hand is rested fully on the part, the superimposed hand rests on top of it either obliquely across when working on the opposite side of the body (Fig. 2.12) or palm over fingers as in Fig. 6.9 when working on the adjacent side of the body. The upper hand must not exert such constant pressure that the kneading by the under hand is distorted. Both hands work together. The body movements of the operator are a forward and backward sway from the feet, to enhance depth, but control must be exerted to prevent the circle of the kneading developing a sharp point at the moment of maximum pressure combined with the movement of the hands as they perform the most distant part of the circle.

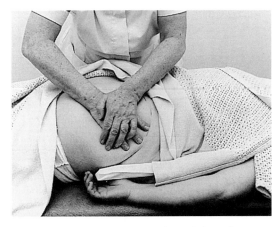

Fig. 2.12 Superimposed (re-inforced) kneading.

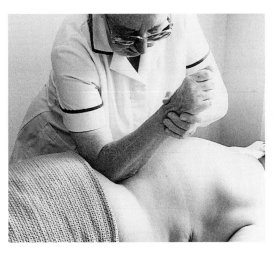

Fig. 2.13 Elbow kneading.

(6) Elbow kneading (for greater depth)

This is performed by the bent elbow which is placed on the area to be treated. The best available part of this elbow is used to form stationary circular manipulations usually on the muscles of the interscapular region and the back or gluteal region where greater depth is required (Fig. 2.13).

(7) Heel of hand kneading (for greater depth)

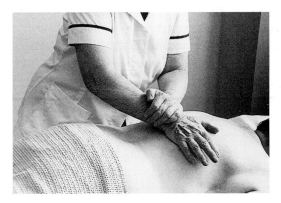

Fig. 2.14 Heel of hand kneading.

The whole heel of the hand is used, being careful not to dig in with the pisiform. This means thin hands may perform painfully. The remainder of the palm and fingers are held off contact and a small circular manipulation is performed. Greater depth can be achieved by reinforcing with the palm of the other hand on top of the working palm or by holding the wrist with the other hand as in Fig. 2.14. This manipulation can be used as an alternative to deep finger and thumb kneading on any well padded area. It is thus useful on muscle bellies but not on tendinous areas where the heel of the hand will 'bounce' across the tendons.

Picking up

Picking up is a manipulation in which the tissues are compressed against underlying bone, then lifted, squeezed and released. The manipulation is more usually performed singlehanded with the thumb and thenar eminence as one component and the medial two or three fingers and hypothenar eminence as the other component of the grasp. The thumb must be opposed and abducted and the degree of these two movements will produce:

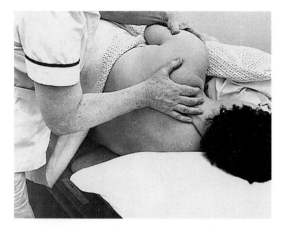

Fig. 2.15 Single-handed kneading.

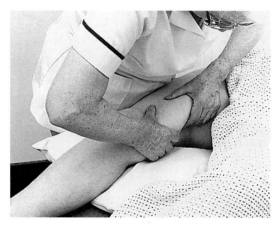

Fig. 2.16 Picking up. The 'C' shape of the hand. Also shows double-handed, alternate work.

either a 'C' shaped grasp (Fig. 2.16) which is wider on larger areas

or a 'V' shaped grasp (Fig. 2.17) which is narrower on areas of lesser bulk.

The cleft between the thumb and index finger should always be in contact with the subject's skin, otherwise a pinching effect is produced and depth is lost. As body weight transfer is important, walk standing is the stance required.

Picking up should be performed with your arms held in slight abduction and with semi-flexed elbows. The wrists are always used initially extended and are more extended as the grasp is effected. Your wrists should never be flexed as this will cause you to pivot on your thumb and finger tips with a screwing action.

Place your hand on the part so that the thumb cleft lies across the centre line of the muscle bulk, with your thumb and thenar eminence disposed on one side and your medial two or three fingers and hypothenar eminence on the other side. Exert compression by transferring your body weight from your feet through your forearm and to the whole hand.

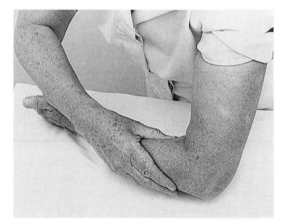

Fig. 2.17 Picking up. The 'V' shape of the hand (practise on own forearm).

Count this as **one**. Then immediately grasp, using the two grasp components equally so that your wrist extends more, but do not further flex any part of your thumb and fingers. This exerts a squeeze, and a simultaneous lift of the tissues will occur. Count this as **two**. Release your grasp – count this as **three**. Your body weight should still be forward, but as you move your relaxed hand on to the next part, maintaining the current conformation, take your body weight back again to your starting position. Count this as **four**. Thus the body weight movement is:

- forward on the count **one**
- backward on the count **four**

while the hand:

- compresses on **one**
- grasps on **two** (lift occurs)
- releases on **three**
- moves on **four**

Learning this combination of movements is one of the more difficult tasks in massage training. Practise first with each hand working backward, down the length of a muscle (Fig. 2.16) or up the length of a muscle. Then try travelling in the reverse direction on the longer muscle masses, as in the lower limb, leading up to working one hand travelling backwards as the other hand travels forwards at such a distance that your fingers and thumbs never touch but the muscle is constantly lifted (Fig. 2.16).

Alternatively, on larger muscle masses such as the anterior aspect of the thigh, your two hands may work as one unit spanning the muscle. Your hands lie so that the thumb of the first hand lies alongside the index finger of the second hand. The thumb of this second hand lies under the heel and alongside the hypothenar eminence of the first hand (Fig. 2.18). The compression is performed by both hands. The grasp is performed by radial extension of both wrists so that the tissues are lifted and squeezed between the medial part of the palms and medial three fingers of both hands. The tissues are released, and your hands move backwards as one unit for one third of their length on to a new area.

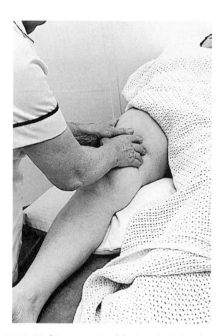

Fig. 2.18 Picking up. Double-handed simultaneous work.

Wringing

Wringing is a manipulation in which the tissues are compressed against the underlying structures prior to lifting them, as in picking up. Then, instead of squeezing the tissues, you pull gently towards yourself with the fingers of one hand while the thumb of your other hand pushes gently in the opposite direction. The tissues are kept elevated and passed from hand to hand by moving the non-pressing component of each hand in turn along the tissues (Fig. 2.19(a)).

The smaller the tissue, the more the tips of your thumbs and fingers are used, and your arms are more adducted and wrists lifted to be more alongside one another. If your arms are abducted and your wrists and forearms lie more parallel with the long axis of the tissues, then the bigger manipulation can be performed.

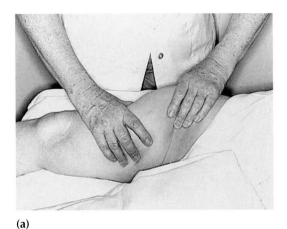

(a)

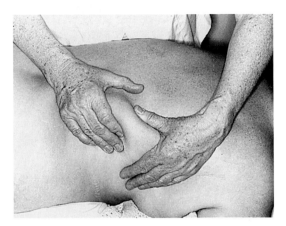

Fig. 2.20 Wringing on superficial tissues.

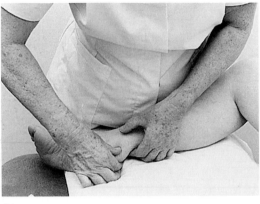

(b)

Fig. 2.19 Wringing: (a) on a muscle belly; (b) on the tendocalcaneous.

Rolling manipulations

The most common rolling manipulation is skin rolling, but muscles may also be rolled.

Skin rolling

Skin rolling is a manipulation in which the skin is lifted and rolled between the thumbs and fingers of the two hands. The manipulation is most often performed on the back, abdomen and thighs but it is also used round superficial joints such as the knee, and in modified form on scar tissue which is shortening and thickening.

Stand in walk standing at the side of the area to be treated and facing across it. Place both hands on the surface of the area more distal from you so that your palms are fully in contact, with your thumb tips touching and parallel to the long axis of the part. Your thumbs should be abducted to such an extent that your index fingers do not touch and indeed should have a space between them (Fig. 2.21).

Maintain full palmar contact and pull your hands backwards towards yourself, without

When the tissue is very small, as in the case of the tendocalcaneus, the manipulation is performed between your thumbs and finger tips as in Fig. 2.19(b). There is an intermediate manner of performance on small muscle groups such as the upper limb muscles. Greater length of your finger pads is used with your thumbs turned so that a greater length of your thumb pad is available on the other side of the muscle tissue. The manipulation may also be performed as a skin wringing, an alternative to skin rolling when only the superficial tissues are lifted and wrung (Fig. 2.20).

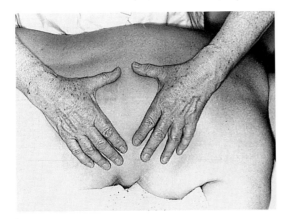

Fig. 2.21 Skin rolling – start.

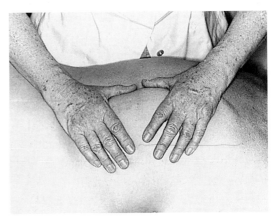

Fig. 2.22 Skin rolling – pull back.

changing their shape and with sufficient pressure to pull the underlying skin (Fig. 2.22). Next, apply pressure with your thumbs as you adduct and oppose them with some depth so that they remain in line with each other but the skin is pushed in a roll towards the fingers (Fig. 2.23). Almost simultaneously, your palms should gradually lift off the skin but your finger tips should remain in contact. Now roll your thumbs forwards still maintaining the roll of skin in your grasp and the skin will roll against your fingers. Your wrists should be flexed and ulnar deviated as this occurs, so that the skin is folded over on top of your fingers (Fig. 2.24).

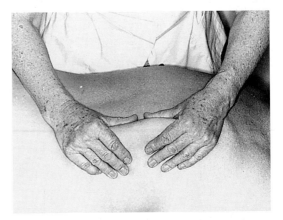

Fig. 2.23 Skin rolling – squeeze and lift.

Try not to 'creep' your fingers as you roll as this can tickle. On adherent skins the skin will only lift slightly and the length of the rolling action must be shortened. The model shown in Figs 2.21–2.24 had very mobile skin and half the width of the back could be treated at once. For adherent skin two or three lines of work should be done instead of the one line shown in Figs 2.21–2.24.

Muscle rolling

Muscle rolling is performed by working across the muscle fibres and along the long axis of

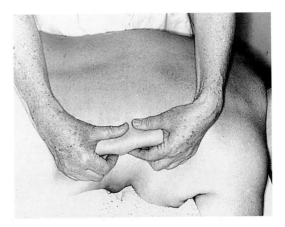

Fig. 2.24 Skin rolling – roll.

muscles. You should be in walk standing to allow weight transference. The lateral boundaries of the muscle should be palpated, then your thumbs placed tip to tip along one border with your fingers along the opposite border (Fig. 2.25). Apply a little pressure with both components so that the muscle bulges slightly between your thumbs and fingers. Then push first with your thumbs and release the pressure simultaneously with the fingers which move to an adjacent area (Fig. 2.25(a)). Rapidly reverse,

pressing with the fingers and releasing the pressure of your thumbs which also move to an adjacent area (Fig. 2.25(b)). It is often a more effective and comfortable manipulation if the pressure is slightly down into the muscle mass rather than back and forth across it. This manipulation can be performed slowly and deliberately to exert a slight stretch, or faster so that there is stimulation to the circulation.

Muscle shaking

All long muscle bellies may be shaken and the manipulation may be performed on the larger muscles such as biceps, triceps, the quadriceps and also on the small muscles of the thenar and hypothenar eminences.

The manipulation is one in which:

For longer muscles the length of your thumb should be placed on one side of the muscle belly and all your fingers placed on the other side of the muscle belly. Your palm should be off-contact (Fig. 2.26). Your hand is then rapidly shaken from side to side as you traverse the length of the muscle belly avoiding contact with

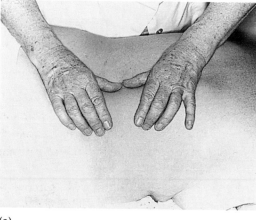

(a)

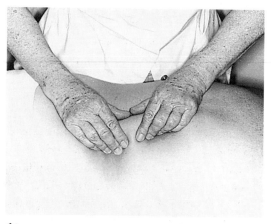

(b)

Fig. 2.25 Muscle rolling: (a) Push with the flat thumbs. (b) Pull back with the finger tips.

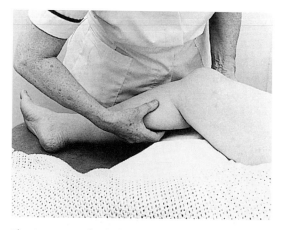

Fig. 2.26 Muscle shaking on the calf muscles.

the underlying bone. Stand in walk standing so that your weight is transferred as you work from proximal to distal on the muscle belly. The muscle will be 'thrown' rapidly from side to side and feels very invigorated.

For very small muscles, the tip of your thumb should be placed on one side, and an appropriate number of finger tips placed on the other side of the muscle belly, and the shaking movement described above is performed.

The friction manipulations

Frictions are small range, deep manipulations performed on specific anatomical structures with the tips of the fingers or thumbs. No other part of the practitioner's hand must rest on the part. There are two types of frictions:

- circular
- transverse

Circular frictions

Circular frictions are performed with the finger tips. The structure to be treated should be identified by careful palpation and the finger tip(s) placed so that they cover the area. The rest of the hand is kept off-contact. Pressure is applied and a small, stationary manipulation is performed, in a circular manner and at gradually increasing depth for three or four circles. The pressure is released and the manipulation is repeated. One hand may reinforce the other on deeper structures. The manipulation can be used over ligaments and myofascial junctions (Fig. 2.27).

Transverse frictions

Transverse frictions were advocated by Dr J. Cyriax in 1941 for treatment of tendon, liga-

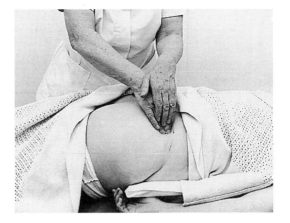

Fig. 2.27 Circular frictions to the attachments on the iliac crest.

ment, myofascial junctions and muscles. The manipulation is performed with:

either the thumb tip
or the finger tip of the index finger sometimes reinforced by placing the tip of the middle finger on top of the index finger nail (Fig. 2.28)
or by the middle finger reinforced by placing the index finger on top of the middle finger nail (more useful when the hand is curved round a limb)
or by two finger tips when a long structure is affected (such as a tendon)
or by the opposed fingers and thumb on structures which can be grasped e.g. tendocalcaneous

Identify the structure to be treated and place your fingers across the longitudinal axis of the structure, i.e. across the length of the collagen fibres (Figs 2.28, 2.29, 2.30, 2.31, 2.32).

Now perform the friction by moving your digit and the model's skin as one, keeping your digit, hand and forearm in a line parallel to the movement to be performed. Do not flex and extend only your digit or wrist. Learn to use

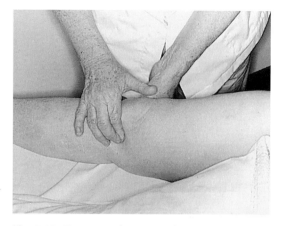

Fig. 2.28 Transverse friction to the medial ligament of the knee.

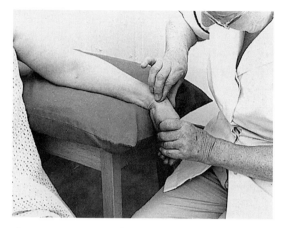

Fig. 2.30 Transverse friction to the tendon sheaths of extensor pollicis longus and abductor pollicis longus.

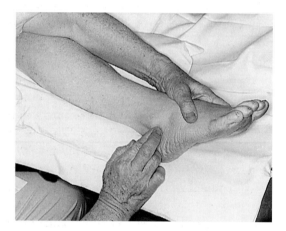

Fig. 2.29 Transverse friction to the lateral ligament of the ankle.

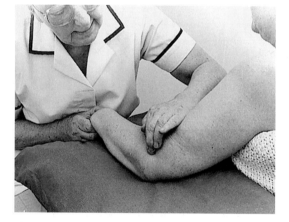

Fig. 2.31 Transverse friction to the common extensor tendon.

both hands so that you lessen your own fatigue. Try to use a movement from your upper arm, trunk or feet so that you achieve greater power with less fatigue. Either sit down or stand in walk standing.

Start to move your fingers forwards and backwards across the structure under treatment with sufficient sweep to produce separation of the fibres at a depth to engage the affected tissue rather than at the patient's tolerance. He or she should be warned that the treatment may be painful, but that numbness may supervene as it progresses. The movement must not take place between your fingers and the model's skin, but between the affected structure and the overlying tissues.

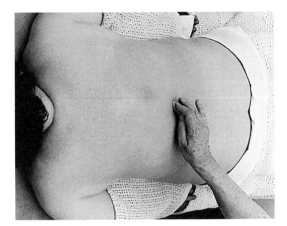

Fig. 2.32 Transverse friction to supraspinous ligament.

The model's skin must be dry to ensure your fingers do not slip. If necessary, apply either spirit or a wisp of cotton wool to the part. The wool is kept in position during the treatment. With these precautions blistering should not occur, but transient redness or slight bruising in adipose tissue may arise.

Maintain the friction for five to ten minutes but the area should be examined at intervals to check that bruising is not occurring or the skin blistering.

Keep tendons taut by putting them on the stretch (Figs 2.30 and 2.31), but keep muscles relaxed by positioning the model so that the part and the attachments of the muscle are approximated during treatment.

Tapôtement or percussive manipulations

The percussive manipulations are those in which the treated part is struck soft blows with the hands. They are performed either to assist evacuation from hollow organs, or to stimulate either skin or muscle reflexes. Stand in walk standing and try practising on a pillow or a padded couch, except for vibrations which may be practised on a partly filled hot water bottle.

The manipulations are:

(1) Clapping
(2) Hacking
(3) Vibrations (shakings)
(4) Beating
(5) Pounding
(6) Tapping

Clapping

Clapping (Figs 2.33, 2.34 and 2.35) is a manipulation in which the whole palmar aspect of the hand is used to strike the body part. The hand is, however, cupped in such a manner that the centre of the hand does not touch the part, but is hollowed. The fingers are slightly flexed, more so at the metacarpophalangeal joints of the index, middle and ring fingers. The thumb is adducted so that it lies just under the index finger and adjacent palm. The hand must be kept in this posture but as relaxed as possible. The wrists should be used to create the difference between striking a hollow sounding blow and a slightly sharper blow. (Slapping sounds very sharp.) The former will have the depth to cause 'jarring' and is used to evacuate hollow organs. The latter is for skin stimulation.

The difference is brought about by the arm movements performed and the effects they have on the hands. The percussive effect is achieved when the heel of the hand is lifted from the part more than the finger tips. The wrist is thus flexed (Fig. 2.33). This movement is brought about by lifting the arm into abduction (beer drinking action when using a tankard) and allowing it to drop. The velocity of the drop

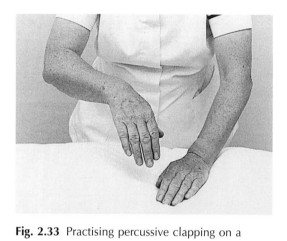

Fig. 2.33 Practising percussive clapping on a pillow.

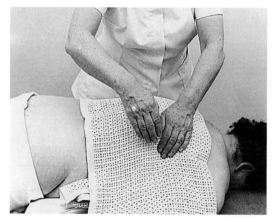

Fig. 2.34 Percussive clapping on the chest.

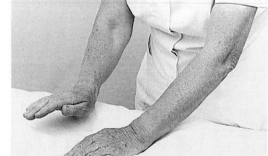

Fig. 2.35 Practising skin stimulating clapping on a pillow.

(not the height) creates the depth of the work. This deeper manipulation is usually performed with the skin lightly covered by a sheet, thin blanket or a single layer of the patient's clothing (Fig. 2.34).

The more stimulating manipulation is also brought about by arm abduction, but with the finger tips raised from the body part without increasing the wrist flexion. In other words the whole hand is raised. The 'strike' is brought about by actively lowering the arm (Fig. 2.35). The tempo of the action should be slower to obtain greater depth, and faster for skin stimulation.

Hacking

Hacking is a manipulation in which the skin is struck using the back of the tips of the three medial fingers. A correct performance is dependent on:

- The initial posture of the whole of the operator's arms and hands with good wrist extension
- A good range of pronation and supination of the radio-ulnar joints

The only movement required is that of pronation and supination. The elbows **must not** flex and extend. The hands are held at a small distance apart so that as they rotate alternately, they just clear one another. The arms are in slight abduction, the elbows are flexed to a right angle with the forearms held parallel with the model's skin and far enough above it to allow only the backs of the little, ring and middle fingers to touch when the forearm is in supination. The wrists are well extended to about 50° (Fig. 2.36).

NB This manipulation cannot be performed properly with less than 50° extension of the wrists. The fingers are in relaxed flexion, i.e.

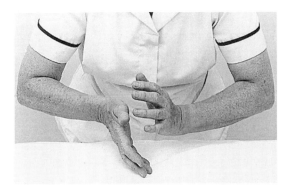

Fig. 2.36 Practising hacking on a pillow.

the posture the relaxed hand adopts spontaneously, and are separated.

Experiment by resting the finger tips of your hands on each other with your little finger resting on the model's skin. Then slightly separate the finger tips – less than 1.5 cm – and check to see if pronation and supination are alternately possible without your finger tips touching those of the other hand.

The 'strike' is modified by the vigour applied to the rotatory movement. A very light hacking produces a susurration, whereas vigorous hacking should sound like a sharp striking noise. Initially, try a slow rate of 10 strikes per five seconds with each hand, then work up to a fast rate of 20–30 strikes per five seconds with each hand. Single strikes can achieve great depth and can be used to obtain reflex contractions of muscle. Slow, deep hacking may produce mechanical effects on hollow organs. All hacking, but especially fast work, produces effects on the skin circulation, and appropriate subjects demonstrate this by producing distinct erythema (reddening) of the skin at the points of strike.

Vibrations

Vibrations are often wrongly called shakings. The difference is that a vibration involves a

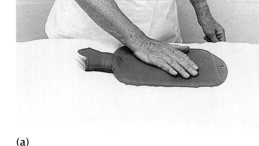

(a)

(b)

Fig. 2.37 Practising vibrations on: (a) a rubber hot water bottle; (b) the abdomen.

movement in which the tissues are pressed and released using an up and down motion. In shaking, the movement on the model is sideways and involves rapid radial and ulnar deviation of your wrists.

Vibrations may be fine or very coarse and demonstrate best on a partly filled rubber hot water bottle or on the abdomen (Fig. 2.37), though the more common use is on the chest.

Vibrations may be performed with the whole hand, or the finger tips. Practise with your hand stationary or slide it backwards and forwards on the area. They are best practised by placing the whole hand on a partly filled hot water bottle with the arm outstretched, and oscillating the whole hand into rapid and minute wrist flexion and extension. The movement is sustained from the shoulder and can be observed to occur spontaneously in some people if the arms are outstretched.

Beating

Beating is a much less used manipulation in which the loosely clenched fist is used for the 'strike'. Its value lies in that the hand is made smaller, but is used as in clapping.

The fingers are flexed at the metacarpophalangeal and proximal interphalangeal joints, but extended at the distal interphalangeal joints so that there is a flat surface composed of the backs of the two distal phalanges and the margin of the palmar surface of the palm. The thumb is kept flat against the lateral part of the flexed hand. The most important part of the operator's action is to raise the whole arm into abduction and allow the wrist to droop (Fig. 2.38) in relaxation. The arm is allowed to drop and strike the part. The speed to attain is six strikes per 10 seconds.

Pounding

Pounding is a less used manipulation but also has value in that it is a form of hacking done with a loosely clenched fist.

The fingers are loosely flexed at all the joints and the thumb lies flat on the lateral side of the hand halfway between adduction and flexion.

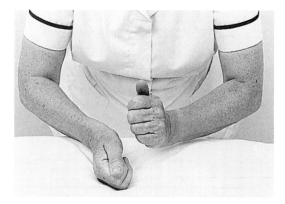

Fig. 2.39 Practising pounding on a pillow.

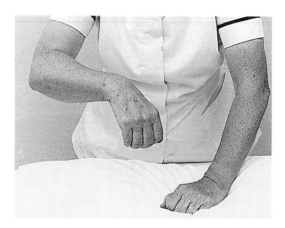

Fig. 2.38 Practising beating on a pillow.

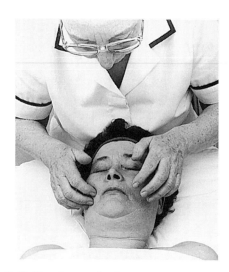

Fig. 2.40 Tapping on the face.

The action is exactly that of hacking, i.e. pronation and supination of the semi-flexed forearms so that the 'strike' is with the knuckles of the little finger (Fig. 2.39). The rate of 'strike' is slightly slower than in hacking.

Tapping

Tapping is performed with the tips of the finger pads and is used on very small areas such as the face (Fig. 2.40). The hand is held relaxed over the area to be treated and the fingers tap at a depth to produce a slightly hollow sound. The index, middle and ring fingers may be used together or in any smaller number, or these three fingers may be used singly in sequence. Both forms of tapping are seen in restless or irritated people who tap chair arms.

Chapter 3
EFFECTS AND CONTRA-INDICATIONS FOR MASSAGE

*Janice M. Warriner and
the late Alison M. Walker*

Observation of the animal kingdom suggests that 'rubbing' of different types is useful to deal with the various discomforts of living. We have all observed domesticated animals 'licking' and 'stroking' wounded areas. Puppies and kittens are licked to facilitate digestive functions. Some primates rub each other to assist toleration of or relieve disorder. Everyone of us has been rubbed or patted in infancy to assist voiding of wind and also to comfort and induce sleep in the fretful. Most of us will have held and then rubbed our bumps and painful areas such as disordered joints and muscles. These are subjective glimpses of some of the perceived benefits that massage may provide.

Massage has been regarded for a long time as having a variety of physiological and psychological effects (if from a largely empirical base). In recent years the therapeutic trend is ever more towards evidence-based practice and this has led to an evergrowing body of research seeking to establish scientifically the effects of massage. The research investigating the effects of massage, as with many areas of medicine, has produced evidence that is incomplete and often contradictory.

The potential effects of massage are many and variations in technique introduce yet another array of variables. Replication of studies is hindered by such subtleties as changes in rhythm or depth of technique and the length of application of massage. Many studies report misleading findings due to methodological problems.

Despite the problems with some of the research into the effects of massage, there would seem to be reasonable consensus with subjectively claimed benefits as to the systems and areas of the body affected by massage. Massage has effects which have been described traditionally under the following main headings:

(1) Mechanical
(2) Physiological
    - on the circulatory system
    - on the nervous system
    - on the musculoskeletal system
(3) Psychological

There is some difficulty in completely separating the effects under these individual headings as it would seem some effects could have appeared under at least two headings; for example circulatory effects on the skin may be viewed as both mechanical and physiological. Part of the problem arises from the fact that massage is a system of mechanical techniques and when applied to living tissues subsequent effects are usually physiological – if at times bordering on the pathophysiological. Few effects would seem to be mechanical only. Subdivision of physiological effects into circulatory and neurological may also be problematic as all discovered effects do not fit neatly into these subheadings.

The effects of massage will be discussed under these main headings, while acknowledging semantic variations.

Mechanical effects

Massage may have a number of effects on the skin. The constant passage of the hands over the skin will remove dead surface cells and allow the sweat glands, the hair follicles and the sebaceous glands to be free of obstruction and to function better. The increased lubricant effect is seen especially when desquamation is a problem. The circulatory effects on the skin are exhibited in some subjects by obvious pinkening and by an increase in warmth often commented on by the patient.

Mobilisation of the skin and tissues at deeper levels is possible through the mechanical influence of the massage. The lightest massage will cause movement of the epidermis by the movement of the hand over the skin. In turn the epidermis moves on the underlying tissues and the dermis on deeper tissues.

Therapeutically, massage has been used widely in the management of scar tissue, the benefits of which can be observed most readily when healing of the skin is involved. Approximately 5 days after any damage has been sustained the weaker type III collagen is laid down as part of the repair process and begins to be converted to the stronger type I collagen (Lakhani *et al.* 1993). Massage may provide externally applied stresses that can influence the conversion of one type of collagen to another as well as the alignment of fibres which tends to be along lines of stress.

The stretching effects of carefully selected massage manipulations can help in promoting or retaining mobility of new 'skin' tissue relative to underlying tissue layers. The mechanical stresses of massage are useful to attempt to counter the tendency for repair scar tissue to shrink and shorten. Massage is often very successful in maintaining scar length while contributing to the strength of the repair and maybe assisting with other changes in the surrounding area even if they are more through circulatory effects.

There is good reason to believe these positive influences on superficial scar tissue can be repeated at deeper tissue levels. Mobility between tissue interfaces occurs normally unless fibrous adhesions are present, when massage may stretch the tissues on one another. Appropriately timed massage intervention to encourage strength and alignment of repair fibres can enhance the natural process of healing in the tissues.

The percussive manipulations performed over the lungs, have the mechanical effect of jerking adherent mucous free from the bronchial tree and, aided by gravity, assisting the removal of sputum towards the upper respiratory passages. The jarring effect and the vibratory effect probably cause some mixing of respiratory gases, while vibrations performed on the distended, wind-laden abdomen cause movement of the wind and relief of discomfort, whether in the infant after a feed, or patients in the post-operative abdominal recovery stage.

Physiological effects

On the circulatory system

When massage is applied to the skin there is quite often an observable change of colour in the area. This change has been attributed most usually to the massage having an effect on the circulatory system. It has been reasonable to consider that massage applied to deeper structures would have similar effects on the blood vessels within such structures. Research papers have attempted to explore many aspects of the circulatory effects achieved by massage. Circulatory flow – venous, lymphatic, arterial – blood velocity and blood viscosity have all been areas of investigation during the last 50 years.

The squeezing, compressive and pushing elements of the massage manipulation carried out with centripetal pressure are widely considered to bring about drainage of venous blood and lymph. This was a view held by Scull (1945) who considered that venous and lymphatic flow could be mechanically enhanced in this way by 'displacement of their contents into regions subjected to lesser pressure'. Scull hypothesised further that such changes in circulatory flow may have occurred due to neuro-vascular adjustments.

A more recent study, by Mortimer *et al.* (1990), looked at skin lymph flow in anaesthetised pigs using a 'hand-held' massager. The researchers found significantly increased (p < 0.005) isotope clearance rates in the massaged leg compared with the contra-lateral leg.

It is difficult to relate these findings directly to the effects of manual massage on the conscious human but it does encourage speculation

as to how changes in venous and lymphatic flow may be achieved.

The drainage of venous blood can be observed if a dependent hand in which the superficial veins are easily observed, is stroked firmly. The soft walled veins are compressed and the blood within them flows onward or centripetally. Its return is stopped by the presence of valves, which prevent backflow, and by the blood behind waiting to take its place. Lymph vessels are also thin walled and affected in the same way. All the minute drainage vessels must be equally affected so that as blood and lymph flows onwards more rapidly due to the massage, the replacing blood moves more quickly. In this way the drainage of treated tissues is enhanced allowing fresh blood an unimpeded flow.

A number of studies have attempted to investigate changes in blood flow and have produced variable findings. Wakim *et al.* (1949) determined blood flow using venous occlusion plethysmography, a technique whereby the arterial flow is calculated from increased limb volume following venous occlusion. Following the application of vigorous, stimulating massage to normal subjects, average increases in blood flow of 57% and 42% for upper (n = 12) and lower (n = 14) extremities respectively were found. Even greater increases averaging 103% were shown following massage of limbs (n = 7) which were flaccidly paralysed following poliomyelitis. However, Wakim states that this massage is more forceful than that normally used by therapists and suggests that such pressure could be damaging to flaccid limbs. No evidence is provided for these assumptions.

In the same paper Wakim also reports findings on blood flow alterations using a less vigorous 'modified Hoffa type of deep stroking and kneading'. In a normal subject no significant increases in blood flow were found. Taking a 15% or above increase as significant

Wakim reported significant increases in four out of six observations of massage to flaccidly paralysed limbs with an average increase of 22% over the six readings.

Similarly, Severini and Venerando (1967) found significant increases in blood flow with deep massage. Only insignificant changes were noted with superficial massage.

In 1952 Ebel and Wisham, using sodium radio-isotope clearance procedures, found no increase in calf muscle blood flow after 10 minutes' massage in comparison with a control test the previous day (n = 7). Hansen and Kristensen (1973), using ^{133}xenon isotope clearance, found a significant increase (p < 0.01) in muscle blood flow during 5 minutes' effleurage. This was followed by a significant decrease (p < 0.05) for 2 minutes post massage before returning to baseline values. The authors hypothesise that increases in blood flow during massage may be due to emptying of the capillary bed, leading to a decrease in blood flow post massage as the capillary bed refills. The authors also comment that the increases are relatively small, even less than in light exercise.

Also using ^{133}xenon clearance as an indicator of muscle blood flow, Hovind and Nielson (1974) compared the effects of 2 minutes' petrissage to thigh and forearm to 2 minutes' tapôtement to the contralateral thigh and forearm (n = 9). Resting values were recorded prior to the intervention. Blood flow significantly increased (p < 0.01) following tapôtement but no significant change was noted following petrissage. The researchers suggest that tapôtement might cause repeated muscular contractions precipitating to increased blood flow.

In a more recent study Tiidus and Shoemaker (1995) measured muscle blood velocity using ultrasound velocimetry (n = 9). Arterial blood velocity was measured before and during a 10 minute massage comprising deep and superficial effleurage, at 1 hour and 72 hours post treatment. Venous blood velocity was measured at 72 hours post treatment. No significant differences were noted between the rest and massage conditions for either arterial or venous velocities.

All these studies are hampered by small sample sizes and the gross nature of the measurements. Studies of the minute circulation to specific areas where the blood flow was compromised by trauma or disease might prove a more useful source of information. Comparison of these findings is difficult due to variations in massage applications and research methods.

Ernst *et al.* (1987) explored the effects of massage on blood viscosity. Using 12 healthy adults, blood viscosities were measured before and after a 20 minute whole body massage. A significant fall (p < 0.05) in native blood viscosity, haematocrit and plasma viscosity was noted. The researchers conclude that such viscosity changes suggest an inflow into the general circulation of low viscosity fluid derived either from stagnant microvessels or from interstitial fluid. Either of these could have therapeutic benefits. However, no control group was included in this study to compare the effects of rest and postural changes alone. The authors do state that they have studied these effects previously and found only small, insignificant falls in viscosity. In opposition to the findings of Ernst, Arkko *et al.* (1983) had previously found no change in haematocrit values following a 1 hour whole body massage.

On a cautionary note, when studying both humans (n = 6) and dogs (n = 8), Eliska and Eliskova (1995) found that massage applied at pressures of 70 to 100 mmHg caused damage to lymphatic vessels. The damage was greater if oedema was present.

Blood pressure, heart rate, skin temperature and conductivity, and oxygen consumption are among the factors researched. The findings of

studies of the effects of massage on these parameters are inconsistent. Comparison of studies
is fraught with difficulties: study groups vary
from the healthy to the critically ill; the massage
applied varied from a one minute back rub to
a one hour whole body massage.

A number of well-designed studies failed to
find significant differences in a variety of physiological measures as a result of massage. However, many of these studies had very small
sample sizes. Some studies found significant
increases while others found significant decreases as a result of massage. A number of
studies continued measurements for some
minutes after massage with variable findings as
to the persistence of the effect. Until large scale
well-controlled studies using similar massage
intervention have been conducted the picture
will remain unclear.

However, it appears unlikely the changes in
blood pressure or heart rate will be great
enough to be of danger to patients. The benefits
of any decrease in blood pressure would only
be of clinical usefulness if the carryover effect
was sufficient. Further studies into this aspect
are required.

The observable effects in the human are
cutaneous circulatory responses occurring in
the following order:

(1) A transient white line appears in response
     to light pressure and is the result of an
     initial capillary constriction.
(2) Because the tissues are slightly trauma-
     tised by most massage manipulations and
     more so by those such as skin rolling and
     the percussive manipulations, a histamine-
     related substance is released.

Histamine is stored in mast cells in the connective tissues, and in the basophil cells and
platelets of blood, all of which may be dis-
turbed or traumatised by the various massage
manipulations. The effect of release of this substance is the triple response which follows. It
involves three reactions which follow each
other rapidly. A red line appears and is caused
by dilatation of the minute blood vessels inde-
pendent of the somatic supply of the skin area.
A flare of redness often described as a 'flush'
then appears around the area and is due to a
widespread dilatation of skin arterioles. This is
brought about by the axon reflex. The third
feature of the triple response is slight swelling
usually described as a wheal. The increased per-
meability of the capillary walls allows escape of
more tissue fluid so that the area becomes
slightly swollen. This fluid is almost identical
with lymph.

On the nervous system

Massage is recognised as having effect on the
nervous system. Different methods of application will provide subtle variations of afferent
input that in turn may cause a number of possible effects. Practice suggests that manipulations need to be selected for specific effects that
they may cause. It is believed that the diamet-
rically opposite effects of sedation or stimulation of a patient may be achieved by selection
of appropriate tempo, degree of pressure and
length of continuity of each manipulation and
the massage as a whole. It is noticeable that the
sedative effect appears to require longer to
achieve than the stimulatory effect, whether
applied to the patient as a whole or to individual parts of the body.

In recent years researchers have begun to
turn their attention to proving some of the
claimed effects. An ever increasing knowledge
of the mechanisms operating within the nervous system has encouraged this research, along
with a revival of interest in massage as a
therapy and the development of suitable means
of measurement.

Alpha motoneuron excitability

A team of researchers from Montreal has carried out a series of studies on the effect of massage on the H-reflex excitability. Hoffman or H-reflex represents an indirect measure of spinal motor neurone excitability and therefore the excitability of the spinal reflex pathway. All these studies, published between 1990 and 1994, have shown consistently a decrease in the H-reflex amplitudes during massage. This denotes a decrease or inhibitory influence on alpha motoneuron excitability. A similar experimental design was used for all the studies: pre-treatment control readings followed by a few minutes massage with readings (individual studies used 3, 4 and 6 minute timings), terminating with post-treatment readings. The triceps surae muscle group was used on each occasion.

Morelli *et al.* (1990), studying nine healthy subjects, were able to demonstrate a 71% decrease in H-reflex amplitude during a 3 minute application of petrissage to the ipsilateral triceps surae, but this amplitude reverted to normal level when the massage was terminated. This suggests that reduced motoneuron excitability occurs only when the massage is being applied and there is no apparent carry-over component. A further study demonstrated that this inhibitory effect is only achieved in the muscle group receiving the petrissage and not in other groups (Sullivan *et al.* 1991).

The study by Morelli *et al.* (1991) using more (20) subjects and a 6 minute period of petrissage confirmed the decreased amplitude of the H-reflex in the triceps surae with still no carry over into the post massage period. However, it went on to exclude factors such as changes in skin temperature, nerve conduction velocity and antagonist activity as being responsible for the decrease in H-reflex excitability. Rapidly adapting cutaneous and/or muscle receptors along with inhibitory poly-synaptic, nonsegmental pathways were proposed by the researchers as possible mediators of the change(s) because of the immediacy of the noted response(s).

In 1992 Goldberg *et al.* showed that reduction of H-reflex excitability occurred with both light petrissage (pressure = 1.25 kPa) and deep petrissage (pressure = 2.5 kPa). A greater effect was noted with deep massage and the research team suggested that pressure sensitive receptors must be implicated in the mechanisms bringing about the inhibition. Sullivan *et al.* (1993) went on to demonstrate that H-reflex excitability could also be decreased during effleurage.

Finally, in 1994 Goldberg *et al.* showed similar reduction in H-reflex amplitude during petrissage of triceps surae in eight out of ten subjects with spinal cord injury. The sample included both complete and incomplete lesions. One complete and one incomplete lesion failed to show the reduced H-reflex amplitude. Despite this the overall results were statistically significant (p = 0.008). The decrease in H-reflex amplitude was not as great and was considered to be less uniform than noted in the subject groups of previous studies. This study did indicate a tendency to some carry-over effect post-massage. Although the sample population was small and this might detract from the finding, it was felt to be 'encouraging' with possible clinical implications if future research could establish this further. Sustained decrease in H-reflex amplitude was not obtained. Massage can be justified as a means of achieving 'temporary' reduction in spinal motoneuron excitability in patients with spinal cord injury, and it can provide a viable option to other accepted treatment techniques.

Pain

Pain is a complex phenomenon of many components and at the very least encompasses physical and emotional elements. There are different types of pain: acute, sharp, fast pain, which is carried to the central nervous system (CNS) along A delta nerve fibres; and chronic, aching, slow pain, which is served by C fibres. Pain is perceived individually and perception thresholds seem to be variable. This variability appears to be found both between individuals and even within a given individual at different times. Pain perception is thought to be under many influences, one of these being afferent input to the CNS. This may be where massage is able to exert its effects.

Control or suppression of pain is deemed to occur at different levels within the nervous system, although mechanisms are still more hypothesis than fully proven (Carreck 1994). Critical key sites for influencing pain are firstly peripheral areas where in the presence of tissue damage, chemical substances such as bradykinin, serotonin and substance P are released and stimulate the free pain receptors (nociceptors) commonly producing the slow pain of injury (Guyton 1992).

The spinal cord is taken to be the next point at which pain may be blocked before signals ascend to the cerebrum for conscious appreciation of the sensation. Since the presentation of the pain gate theory of Melzack and Wall in 1965 and subsequent modifications to this, there has been a basis for believing that sensory traffic, into the dorsal grey areas of spinal cord segments, is sifted and sorted. This is by the complex neuronal circuitry, especially including that within the substantia gelatinosa. Signals from different sources are carried along fibres of different diameters and compete across the synapses of the circuitry, for which signals will have the right to further transmission. Input of signals along large diameter fibre pathways competes with pain signals along smaller diameter fibre pathways and can close the 'pain' gate. This occurs via various influences on synapses – preventing pain signals from further transmission to conscious level. Higher levels of the CNS are considered to be involved in pain control, most probably involving descending pathways and release of endogenous opiate substances.

Some of the descending fibres are thought to emanate from areas such as the brainstem reticular formation and are triggered by certain pain signals reaching that level of the CNS. Some of the subsequent endogenous opiate release will be at the reticular formation and at higher levels but also at spinal cord level and it is suggested this will result in the suppression of pain signals entering at these sites (Holey & Cook 1997).

It has been put forward that the setting of the pain gate is by higher centres and this can dominate neural activity at spinal cord level (Melzak & Wall 1988, cited in Carreck 1994). It is difficult to define with certainty exactly which higher centres may be involved but parts of the cerebral cortex and limbic system have been implicated (Holey & Cook 1997).

Massage may contribute in some way to pain control at all the indicated levels and therefore may influence pain perception and its threshold. Pain receptors are not readily adaptive (Guyton 1992) so if harmful chemicals are present as a result of injury, pain signals are likely to be triggered and carried to the CNS. Massage, used appropriately in accessible peripheral areas of damage, has been observed as having a positive effect in reducing pain. It is speculated that under these circumstances the massage may have altered the local circulation in such a way as to reduce or remove noxious substances thereby reducing or removing stimuli reflected in a corresponding reduction of response by the pain receptors.

Massage can provide the CNS with afferent input, some along the larger diameter A beta fibres, that will compete with incoming pain signals to the spinal cord. This input if of adequate level may block pain signals by a process of presynaptic inhibition and may reduce or prevent transmission to conscious level.

Massage input relative to the higher centres and endogenous opiate release is a somewhat hypothetical area. It may be possible that sensory signals triggered by certain massage techniques stimulate higher levels of the CNS. These areas may be those capable of sending descending signals and this may result in opiate release; some in turn afford pain control through post synaptic inhibition at spinal level. Quite how the highest levels of the CNS are involved is hard to assess. Can they influence brainstem areas or other areas within the cerebrum? How is this influence exerted via opiate release? Can these areas be affected by sensory input from massage and is this the cross-over point with what has been labelled the psychological effect in times past?

Research studies into the relationship of massage and pain control have produced some very mixed results. Some of the studies have examined normals, i.e. subjects without pain, and lead one to wonder if responses are inclined to be different in normals compared with those found in subjects already experiencing pain.

Day *et al.* (1987) chose to investigate the effect of massage on endogenous opiates within the peripheral venous blood. The study consisted of 21 healthy adult volunteers. One group rested for 40 minutes and the other group received 30 minutes back massage using mineral oil. Venous beta endorphin and beta liptropin were measured pre and post treatment. Massage in this set of circumstances did not change the levels of the endogenous opiates. The researchers recommended that a follow-up study using subjects with acute and chronic back pain might give different results. Massage and endogenous opiate release was still considered as the possible mechanism of pain relief.

Weinrich and Weinrich (1990) investigated the effect of massage on patients with cancer pain. The main significant positive finding was a decrease of pain immediately post massage, but only for the male subjects. There were a number of problems with this study. Only 10 minutes back massage was performed by student nurses after a minimal training period of 1 hour. The control group subjects were simply visited by the data collector for 10 minutes. The researchers felt that where there was significant pain reduction this had tended to occur in male subjects already experiencing higher levels of pain than the female subjects, and males within the control group. Pain levels were self reported. This pilot study posed many questions, these largely remaining unanswered. It was considered that massage may be a useful option for short term pain relief.

Puustjarvi *et al.* (1990) investigated 21 female subjects with chronic tension headaches. Each subject received 10 sessions of upper body massage – kneading and stroking with prolonged work over trigger points. Pain measured by questionnaire and visual analogue scale decreased and the number of days with neck pain decreased in the follow-up period at 3 and 6 months. Additionally cervical movements improved, and reduced EMG activity was shown in the frontalis muscle. The researchers felt the study confirmed positive clinical and physiological effects of massage.

Carreck (1994) explored the pain perception threshold of 40 healthy subjects, using 15 minutes of lower limb massage with 20 subjects and 15 minutes rest with the other 20 subjects. Transcutaneous electrical stimulation was used to elicit the point at which subjects first perceived pain. The results showed increased pain perception thresholds in the group who had received massage and it was concluded that massage is a valuable option in management of pain.

Massage and pain will be reviewed further under the musculoskeletal and psychological headings.

On the musculoskeletal system

The focus in this section will be towards the possible effects massage may have on muscles. Inevitably there will be some reference again to pain as muscular pain and soreness are not uncommon.

In a 1989 study by Balke *et al.* researchers investigated how massage might affect muscle fatigue. Subjects performed a gradual exercise test on a treadmill and this was then followed by either rest, or manual or mechanical massage of the legs for about 15 minutes. Exercise performance was re-tested and this improved in both the manual and mechanical massage groups. The sample group was very small but the researchers considered that massage assisted recuperation from fatigue 'more effectively than total rest alone'. This finding is reinforced in a small way by another study investigating a number of modalities with respect to treatment of subacute low back pain. Incorporated in their procedures was the Sorensen fatigue test, which examined trunk extension and how long this might be maintained in seconds to the point of fatigue. Subjects in the massage grouping received 15 minutes' back massage three times per week over a period of 3 weeks. The massage group showed the greatest improvement in best extension effort and fatigue time when compared with the other modalities used such as corset, spinal manipulation (Pope *et al.* 1994).

A 1990 study investigated percussive vibratory massage on short term recovery from muscle fatigue. The experimental group received 4 minutes' percussive vibratory massage and 1 minutes' rest compared with 5 minutes' rest only for the control group. The procedures for the two groups were interspersed between three periods of exercise and rate of fatigue measurements. It was found that there was no significant benefit from massage in the terms of these study conditions. The length of massage time, the type of massage and the timing of the intervention could all be questioned; however, it does not convincingly negate the use of massage for the effects on muscle under different circumstances (Cafarelli *et al.* 1990).

A 1995 cross-over study (Rinder & Sutherland 1995) was more positive about the effect of massage on muscle fatigue. Subjects were exercised to the point of fatigue and on one occasion allotted to the massage group and on the next occasion to the rest group. Massage in the form of effleurage and petrissage was applied for 3 minutes to this fatigued quadriceps muscle. Other subjects rested for 6 minutes. Following immediately after either massage or rest, subjects were asked to complete as many leg extensions as possible against their individual half load maximum. The results showed that massage had significantly improved quadriceps performance compared to rest. The discussion of this study points out that even where no significant effect of massage was elicited, no study has found detrimental effects of massage on muscle fatigue. It also considered that all effects might not be of a purely physical nature and psychological factors could not be ruled out.

Delayed onset muscle soreness (DOMS) can occur in any individual who performs some unaccustomed exercise. It is considered to appear 8–24 hours post exercise, building to its height of discomfort at about 48 hours post exercise and resolving over a few days (Smith *et al.* 1994). DOMS may present as slight discomfort localised to myotendinous areas, to stiffness and extreme pain throughout the muscle. It commonly occurs in association with eccentric muscle activity. It is thought that such activity sets up an acute inflammatory reaction in the muscle and massage intervention may be able to moderate the injury response. Two 1994 studies examined this area, producing variable findings. Smith believed that massage applied 2 hours after exercise could hinder the delivery of neutrophils to the 'injury site', i.e. the exercised muscle, and so reduce the inflammatory response and resultant soreness. Fourteen untrained male subjects exercised elbow flexors and extensors isokinetically and eccentrically. The experimental group was given 30 minutes 'athletic' massage 2 hours post exercise. The control group was rested. DOMS, creatine kinase and neutrophil levels were assessed before exercise and at intervals up to 120 hours post exercise. It appeared that massage reduced DOMS and creatine kinase levels. It produced prolonged elevation of circulating neutrophils leading to the assumption that these had not accumulated in the muscle so the inflammatory response and subsequent soreness were reduced (Smith *et al.* 1994).

The second study by Weber *et al.* (1994) examined DOMS from a slightly different perspective. Muscle soreness and force deficits following high intensity eccentric exercise were investigated using 40 untrained female subjects. These were randomly assigned to one of four groups – therapeutic massage, upper body ergonomics, micro current electrical stimulation or control which took the form of 8 minutes' rest. Soreness was measured using a visual analogue scale. Maximum voluntary isometric contraction (at 90° elbow flexion) and peak torque were assessed using a Cybex isokinetic dynometer. Readings were taken before exercise and at 24 and 48 hours post exercise. The elbow flexors were eccentrically exercised to exhaustion. The massage group were given 2 minutes' light effleurage, 5 minutes' petrissage followed by 1 minute's effleurage immediately

after exercise and after 24 hours at reassessment. No differences were noted between the massage and other groups. The results from this study do not support the use of massage immediately post exercise or 24 hours after exercise to relieve DOMS or the force deficits associated with it.

Some earlier research studies have also produced contradictory findings but often studies are not comparing like with like. There are great variations in types of massage used and length of time it is applied. There is much work to be done to refine study design and consistency. Maybe then tangible proof of the effects of massage will be found.

Muscle tension can lead to pain and soreness. Massage has been used to promote relaxation of muscle and is a means of dealing with or off-setting the development of such discomfort. An early study postulated that tension in muscles on the posterior aspect of the trunk and lower limbs would limit trunk forward flexion. The flexion was measured on a fingers to floor basis. Measurements were taken before and after a 30 minute rest period, before and after a 30 minute massage. The massage was to the whole of the back and lower limbs. All 25 study subjects showed gain in trunk flexibility after undergoing massage compared to the pre and post rest readings. It was concluded that massage can create relaxation in voluntary muscles although mechanisms were not clear. Comment was made that almost all subjects reported a feeling of relaxation and this may implicate higher centre nervous activity relative to spinal circuitry. Local vascular metabolic changes were also proposed as possible contributors (Nordschav & Bierman 1962).

Danneskiold-Samsoe *et al.* (1982) studied 13 women with regional back and shoulder(s) muscle pain and tension. Subjects were given a course of 10 massage treatments each lasting between 30 and 45 minutes. After each massage, plasma myoglobin and the extent of the area of muscle tension were measured. Plasma myoglobin levels rose, following the early massage treatments, reaching a peak some 3 hours after the treatment. It was noted that as muscle tension declined with further treatments, so did the plasma myoglobin levels. The researchers concluded that release of plasma myoglobin occurs from muscles that exhibit tension and that massage assists in the normalisation of muscle tension. Plasma myoglobin showed no change from normal levels when muscles without pain or tenderness were massaged. It suggests that regional muscle tension and pain may be due to disorders of muscle fibres rather than involvement of connective tissue. Mechanisms for these findings were not forthcoming.

This brief survey of some of the available research on the effects of massage on muscles had identified both positive and negative findings.

Psychological effects

A question that comes to mind under this heading is, does this warrant a separate section or are the effects to be discussed just an extension of physiology? Much debate would be possible but the included contents are considered to be either psychological or psychophysiological. Research papers to date have not been very successful in clarifying such matters as it is suggested that much evidence is based on 'anecdotal testimony and practical field experiences' as to the 'positive effects of massage on psychological wellbeing' (Cafarelli & Flint 1992).

An interesting study by Weinberg & Kolodny (1988) investigated the relationship between exercise, massage and mood enhancement. The subjects were 183 students of physical education and they were divided between six groups. These groups were swimming, jogging, racquetball, tennis, a control rest condition and a massage (full body) condition group. The psychological measurement tools used were the profile of mood states (POMS) after McNair (1971), the state anxiety inventory (SAI) of Spielberger (1970), and the Thayer adjective checklist (1967), all cited in Weinberg & Kolodny (1988).

The POMS questionnaire is used to measure mood fluctuations. It contains six subscales: tension–anxiety (somatic tension), depression–dejection (feelings of personal inadequacy), anger–hostility (feelings of intense overt anger), vigour-activity (mood of high energy), fatigue–inertia (mood of weariness and low energy) and confusion–bewilderment (cognitive inefficiency).

The SAI questionnaire is designed to assess the state of anxiety. Thayer's adjective checklist is used to examine anxiety and activation, these recognised respectively through the subscales of high activation (feelings of tension and anxiety) and general activation (feelings of calm and relaxation).

Each subject completed these questionnaires prior to and immediately after their 30 minute period of either exercise, Swedish massage or rest. The results showed that the massage and the running groups were consistently more related to positive mood states and psychological wellbeing immediately after the 'activity'. However it was noted that the benefits were much more marked in the post massage group.

Results from the other groupings generally did not produce significant change. All the subscales of the POMS questionnaire, except the vigour subscale, showed a positive relationship to massage. The beneficial relationship was also demonstrated with regard to the high activation and general activation subscales of Thayer's adjective checklist. The researchers concluded that massage 'consistently related to transitory positive mood enhancement' and psychological wellbeing even if only demonstrated in the setting of the study. It would seem to go part way to justifying subjective comments often made post massage, on its use in the sports context as well as in many other areas of life.

The tension–anxiety part of mood states has been investigated in a number of studies. Some studies have also attempted to link changes in psychological state to altered physiology. Many different subject groups have been used and findings have been of infinite variety. It appears almost easier to assess mood–psychological state changes by the different, available inventories, than to predict physiological responses relative to those changes in psychological dynamics.

Different markers are used to monitor physiological changes. These are commonly blood pressure (systolic and diastolic), heart rate, skin temperature (often of the fingers), galvanic skin response, respiratory rate, saliva composition and somatic electromyography on muscles like the masseter and trapezius, which are often identified as having high levels of tension. There is thought to be much inter-relationship between the continuum of arousal-relaxation and levels of anxiety. High levels of arousal may occur in emotionally stressful situations and often, but not always, this manifests as raised levels of blood pressure, heart rate, EMG activity and constriction of blood vessels in peripheral circulation as demonstrated by reduction of temperature in the fingers (Longworth 1982). Some of these physiological changes will undoubtedly involve adjustments via the autonomic nervous system (ANS).

The following is a brief sampling of studies that have dealt with psychophysiological effects and massage.

Longworth (1982) investigated the effects of slow stroke back massage (SSBM) in 'normo-tensive females' who were nursing students and staff with an age range from 19 to 52 years. This quite complex study attempted to monitor many changes. Anxiety was assessed by use of the state (trait) anxiety inventory of Spielberger, as mentioned previously. A number of physiological readings were taken. Six minutes of uninterrupted slow stroke massage was administered during the approximately 27 minute experimental period, which also contained baseline rest and final rest periods. At the end of the experimental period subjects generally stated they felt rested and relaxed. The researcher believed that the SSBM had been successful in lowering the psycho-emotional and somatic arousal level of subjects into the rest period post massage. This finding was reinforced by significant decreases in SAI scores, demonstrating reduction in anxiety state. It was also noted during the period that EMG levels were reduced, indicating lower levels of muscle tension.

Changes in other physiological markers were more difficult to explain. No significant differences were noted for systolic/diastolic blood pressure or heart rate between the baseline rest and final rest periods of experimental time. It was assumed the massage between the rest periods produced no prolonged effect on the autonomic nervous system even though changes had occurred during the experimental time, e.g. initial rise in systolic blood pressure during the first 3 minutes of massage, and increased heart rate in the last 3 minutes of the 6 minute massage.

A study by Barr & Taslitz (1970) examined the effects of back massage on autonomic functions in 19 college students aged 19–21 years. Each student underwent three massage sessions of 20 minutes with pre and post massage rest periods and three separate control periods of corresponding duration. Some of the physiological findings correspond to those of the

Longworth study and others do not. Heart rate did tend to increase during massage; however, systolic and diastolic blood pressure decreased during the initial period of massage, the latter apparently conflicting with the Longworth findings. Barr considered that back massage did have influence on autonomic functions, mainly an increase on sympathetic activity and a smaller effect on parasympathetic action. It was speculated further whether the changes were primarily as a result of the massage or the mental state of the subjects. This highlights again the mysterious inter-relationships of higher centre activity in the CNS to autonomic adjustments and pain control. What influence do changes of mood or emotions play in physiological adjustments? Does the afferent input of massage change activity in the limbic system, the subcortical and even the cortical areas and do they in turn instigate changes within body systems? Some consistency does appear to be present in the literature regarding the positive effects of massage on mood–anxiety levels in a range of people.

Ferrell-Torry & Glick (1993) investigated whether massage could modify anxiety and the perception of cancer pain as well as monitoring other physiological changes. The study group were nine hospitalised males all experiencing cancer pain. Pain was measured by visual analogue scale and anxiety by Spielberger's state anxiety inventory, these being used before and immediately after massage. Thirty minutes' effleurage, petrissage and myofascial trigger point massage therapy was applied to neck, back and shoulders. Respiratory, heart rates and blood pressure were measured. Massage produced significant reductions in both pain perception (mean 60%) and anxiety (mean 24%) levels. Feelings of relaxation were enhanced. In this study the physiological measures tended to decrease following massage.

Meek (1993) working with 30 hospice clients used SSBM to achieve relaxation. The duration of the massage was only for 3 minutes. Modest but not very prolonged decreases took place in blood pressure and heart rate along with a rise in skin temperature. The researcher took these to be indicative of increased relaxation, which usually means a low arousal level and this suggests low anxiety state (Meek 1993; Longworth 1982).

Groer *et al.* (1994) studied anxiety levels and took post massage saliva samples in a group of 18 well older adults. The control group underwent a 10 minute period of relaxed lying and the experimental group had a 10 minute back rub. SAI questionnaires were completed before and after the intervention. Anxiety levels went down for both the experimental and the control group but not to significant levels. The saliva in the post massage group showed increased levels of immunoglobulin A. This finding is part of a claim that massage can have beneficial effects on the body's immune system. It is not clear why reduction in anxiety did not reach significant levels on this occasion.

Fraser & Ross (1993) also looked at the effect of back massage on elderly residents in institutionalised care. A similar format of monitoring physiological markers, blood pressure, etc. and anxiety levels via Spielberger's self evaluation questionnaire were used pre and post intervention. Three experimental subject groups were given either back massage with normal conversation, conversation only or no intervention. Post test scores were all lower in the massage group although not statistically significant; however, there was a statistically significant difference in mean anxiety score between the massage group and the no intervention group. Verbally subjects reported the back massage to be relaxing. It was felt massage as a form of touch was valuable in care of the elderly person and perhaps assisted communication.

Corley *et al.* (1995) also looked at the effect of back rubs on elderly reidents in care. Mood was found to improve in both massage and rest control groups but not to significant levels. Subjectively the residents commented positively on the back rub. Little of significance was found in physiological measures.

Much of the above reinforces the practice of massage but fully supportive research evidence is as yet elusive.

Snyder *et al.* (1995) looked at the use of hand massage in decreasing agitation behaviours associated with care activities in elderly patients with dementia. Behaviours had been observed for 5 days before massage intervention and 5 days after a 10 day intervention period. There was observed to be some reduction in agitation behaviours such as screaming and punching relative to morning care activities. It was speculated that massage might have achieved the limited effect through bringing a degree of calmness and relaxation to patients' stress levels. This area of study was complicated and much was unexplained.

At the other end of the age spectrum, touch and massage have been examined for effect on children and adolescents. Some of those effects are taken to be psychological. Ottenbacher *et al.* (1987) reviewed 19 studies on the effects of tactile stimulation on infants and young children. Results were variable and dependent on study design, but it was acknowledged that infants and young children respond to tactile stimulation. Performance in such activities as vocalisation and motor skills were much better than in the control or comparison group.

Field *et al.* (1993) looked at anxiety and mood in 52 hospitalised, depressed and adjustment disordered children and adolescents. One grouping had 30 minutes' back massage over 5 days and the other group watched relaxing videotapes. The massage group showed immediate decreased anxiety measured by state anxiety inventory for children (STAIC) questionnaires which were administered before and immediately post treatment. Depressed subjects showed longer term improvement. Using the POMS scores of both depressed and adjustment disordered subjects a less depressed mood was noted by day five. Saliva cortisol noticeably decreased during the massage only. This is usually an indication of lowered arousal and anxiety level.

Two different studies have produced findings regarding changing saliva composition relative to massage when used to create relaxation or reduce anxiety level.

Green and Green (1987) comment that stress is known to be immuno-suppressive, but how enhancing to the immune system is relaxation? Massage to the back (20 minutes) was one of the study groupings and in the post test readings immunoglobulin A was increased.

Ironsen *et al.* (1995) in their study of 29 gay men (20 HIV-positive and 9 HIV-negative), discovered that following a daily massage lasting 45 minutes and given for a month, there were significant decreases in anxiety level and stress hormone levels. Salivary cortisol demonstrated such a decrease. Improvement occurred in immune defence mechanisms, including significant increase in natural killer cell numbers, but no change was noted in HIV disease progression markers.

The research papers that have been reviewed demonstrate some difficulty in attaining consistency of findings. Massage does appear to produce positive and beneficial responses, or no significant response, rather than having any detrimental effects.

The words of Pemberton (1950), cited in Rinder & Sutherland (1995), sum up this chapter thus justifying the continued use of massage: 'successful forms of treatment often run ahead of precise knowledge of the premises from which they arise'.

Contra-indications

Massage is contra-indicated in the following circumstances:

(1)   Skin disorders which would be irritated by either increase in warmth of the part or by the lubricants which might be used, e.g. eczema.
      When superficial infections are suppurating.
(2)   In the presence of malignant tumours.
(3)   Early bruising – though at about the fourth day massage will be of use in treating a haematoma.
(4)   In the presence of recent, unhealed scars or open wounds.
(5)   Adjacent to recent fracture sites and especially at the elbow or mid-thigh.
(6)   Over joints or other tissues which are acutely inflamed, especially joints with tubercular infections.

References

Arkko, P.J., Pakarinen, A.J. & Kar-Koskinen, O. (1983) Effects of whole body massage on serum protein, electrolyte and hormone concentrations, enzyme activities and hematological parameters. *International Journal of Sports Medicine*, (4), 265–7.

Balke, B., Anthony, J. & Wyatt, F. (1989) The effects of massage treatment on exercise fatigue. *Clinical Sports Medicine*, 1, 189–96.

Barr, J.S. & Taslitz, N. (1970) The influence of back massage on autonomic functions. *Physical Therapy*, 50(12), 1679–91.

Cafarelli, E., Sim, J., Carolan, B. & Liebesman, J. (1990) Vibratory massage and short–term recovery from muscular fatigue. *International Journal of Sports Medicine*, (11), 474–8.

Cafarelli, E. & Flint, F. (1992) The role of massage in preparation for and recovery from exercise. *Sports Medicine*, 14(1), 1–9.

Carreck A. (1994) The effect of massage on pain perception threshold. *Manipulative Therapist*, 26(2), 10–16.

Corley, M.C., Ferriter, J., Zeh, J. & Gifford, C. (1995) Physiological and psychological effects of back rubs. *Applied Nursing Research*, 8(1), 39–43.

Danneskiold-Samsoe, B., Christiansen, E., Lund, B. & Andersen, R.B. (1982) Regional muscle tension and pain ('fibrositis'), effect of massage on myoglobin in plasma. *Scandinavian Journal of Rehabilitation Medicine*, 15, 17–20.

Day, J.A., Mason, R.R. & Chesrown, S.E. (1987) Effect of massage on serum level of B-endorphin and B-lipotropin in healthy adults. *Physical Therapy*, 67(6), 926–30.

Ebel, A. & Wisham, L.H. (1952) Effect of massage on muscle temperature and radiosodium clearance. *Archives of Physical Medicine*, July, 399–405.

Eliska, O. & Eliskova, M. (1995) Are peripheral lymphatics damaged by high pressure manual massage? *Lymphology*, 28, 21–30.

Ernst, E., Matrai, A., Magyarosy, I., Liebermeister, R.G.A. *et al.* (1987) Massage cause changes in blood fluidity. *Physiotherapy*, 73(1), 43–5.

Ferrell-Torry, A.T. & Glick, O.J. (1993) The use of therapeutic massage as a nursing intervention to modify anxiety and the perception of cancer pain. *Cancer Nursing*, 16(2), 93–101.

Field, T., Morrav, C., Valdeon, C., Larson, S. *et al.* (1993) Massage reduces anxiety in child and adolescent psychiatric patients. *International Journal of Alternative and Complementary Medicine*, July, 23–27.

Fraser, J. & Ross, J. (1993) Psychophysiological effects of back massage on elderly institutionalized patients. *Journal of Advanced Nursing*, 18, 238–45.

Goldberg, J., Sullivan, S.J. & Seaborne, D.E. (1992) The effect of two intensities of massage on H-reflex amplitude. *Physical Therapy*, 72(6), 449–57.

Goldberg, J., Seaborne, D.E., Sullivan, S.J. & Leduc, B.E. (1994) The effect of therapeutic massage on

H-reflex amplitude in persons with a spinal cord injury. *Physical Therapy*, 74(8), 728–37.

Green, R.G. & Green, M.L. (1987) Relaxation increases salivary immunoglobulin A. *Psychological Reports*, 61, 623–9.

Groer, M., Mozingo, J., Droppleman, P., Davis, M. *et al.* (1994) Measures of salivary suretory immunoglobulin A and state anxiety after a nursing back rub. *Applied Nursing Research*, 7(1), 2–6.

Guyton, A.C. (1992) *Human Physiology and Mechanisms of Disease*. W.B. Saunders Company Limited, Philadelphia.

Hansen, T.I. & Kristensen, J.H. (1973) Effect of massage, shortwave diathermy and ultrasound upon Xe disappearance rate from muscle and subcutaneous tissue in the human calf. *Scandinavian Journal of Rehabilitation Medicine*, (5), 179–82.

Holey E. & Cook, E. (1997) *Therapeutic Massage*. W.B. Saunders Company Limited, London.

Hovind, H. & Nielsen, S.L. (1974) Effect of massage on blood flow in skeletal muscle. *Scandinavian Journal of Rehabilitation Medicine*, (6), 74–7.

Ironsen, G., Field, T., Scafidi, F., Hashimoto, M. *et al.* (1995) Massage therapy is associated with enhancement of the immune system's cytotoxic capacity. *International Journal of Neuroscience*, 1–13.

Lakhani, S.R., Dilly, S.A. & Finlayson, C.J. (1993) *Basic Pathology – an introduction to the mechanisms of disease*. Edward Arnold, London.

Longworth, J.C.D. (1982) Psychophysiological effects of slow back massage in normotensive females. *Advances in Nursing Science*, 4, 44–61.

Meek, S.S. (1993) Effects of slow stroke back massage on relaxation in hospice clients. *Image: Journal of Nursing Scholarship*, 25(1), 17–21.

Morelli, M., Seaborne, D.E. & Sullivan, S.J. (1990) Changes in H-reflex amplitude during massage of triceps surae in healthy subjects. *Journal of Orthopaedic & Sports Physical Therapy*, 12(2), 55–9.

Morelli, M., Seaborne, D.E. & Sullivan, S.J. (1991) H–reflex modulation during manual muscle massage of human triceps surae. *Archives of Physical Medicine and Rehabilitation*, 72(October), 915–19.

Mortimer, P.S., Simmonds, R., Rezvani, M., Robbins, M. *et al.* (1990) The measurement of skin lymph flow by isotope clearance – reliability, reproducibility, injection dynamics, and the effect of massage. *The Journal of Investigative Dermatology*, 95(6), 677–82.

Nordschav, M. & Bierman, W. (1962) The influence of manual massage on muscle relaxation: effect on trunk flexion. *Journal of the American Physical Therapy Association*, 42, 653–7.

Ottenbacher, K.J., Muller, L., Brandt, D., Heintzelman, A. *et al.* (1987) The Effectiveness of Tactile Stimulation as a form of Early Intervention: A Quantitive Evaluation. *Development and Behavioural Paediatrics*, 8(2), 68–76.

Pope, M.H., Reed, B., Phillips, D.C., Haugh, L.D. *et al.* (1994) A prospective randomized three week trial of spinal manipulation, transcutaneous muscle stimulation, massage and corset in the treatment of subacute low back pain. *Spine*, 19(22), 2571–7.

Puustjarvi, K., Airaksinen, O. & Pontinen, P.J. (1990) The effect of massage in patients with chronic tension headache. *International Journal of Acupuncture and Electrotherapeutics*, 13, 159–62.

Rinder, A.N. & Sutherland, C.J. (1995) An investigation of the effects of massage on quadriceps performance after exercise fatigue. *Complementary Therapies in Nursing and Midwifery*, 1, 99–102.

Scull, C.W. (1945) Massage – physiologic basis. *Archives of Physical Medicine*, March, 159–67.

Severini, V. & Venerando, A. (1967) Effect of massage on peripheral circulation and physiological effects of massage. *Europa Medicophysica*, 3, 165–83.

Smith, L.L., Keating, M.N., Holbert, D., Spratt, D.J. *et al.* (1994) The effects of athletic massage on delayed onset muscle soreness, creatine kinase, and neutrophil count: a preliminary report. *Journal of Orthopaedic & Sports Physical Therapy*, 19(2), 93–9.

Snyder, M., Egan, E.C. & Burns, K.R. (1995) Efficacy of hand massage in decreasing agitation behaviours associated with care activities in persons with dementia. *Geriatric Nursing*, 16(2), 60–63.

Sullivan, S.J., Williams, L.R.T., Seaborne, D.E. & Morelli, M. (1991) Effects of massage on alpha motoneuron excitability. *Physical Therapy*, **71**(8), 555–9.

Sullivan, S.J., Seguin, S., Seaborne, D.E. & Goldberg, J. (1993) Reduction of H-reflex amplitude during the application of effleurage to the triceps surae in neurologically healthy subjects. *Physiotherapy Theory and Practice*, 9, 25–31.

Tiidus, P.M. & Shoemaker, J.K. (1995) Effleurage massage, muscle blood flow and long-term post-exercise strength recovery. *International Journal of Sports Medicine*, **16**, 478–83.

Wakim, K.G., Martin, G.M., Terrier, J.C., Elkins, E.C. *et al.* (1949) The effects of massage on the circulation in normal and paralysed extremi-ties. *Archives of Physical Medicine*, March, 135–44.

Weber, M.D., Servedio, F.J. & Woodall, W.R. (1994) The effects of three modalities on delayed onset muscle soreness. *Journal of Orthopaedic & Sports Physical Therapy*, **20**(5), 236–42.

Weinberg, R.J.A. & Kolodny, J. (1988) The relationship of massage and exercise to mood enhancement. *The Sport Psychologist*, **2**, 202–11.

Weinrich, S.P. & Weinrich, M.C. (1990) The effect of massage on pain in cancer patients. *Applied Nursing Research*, **3**(4), 140–45.

Chapter 4
MASSAGE TO THE UPPER LIMB

The whole upper limb is usually treated as one unit. It is so much smaller than the lower limb that it is possible to work all the way down the limb performing the same manipulation in sequence.

Preparation of the model

Ask the model to remove all clothing from the appropriate arm and shoulder. Shoulder straps should also be slipped off.

For a treatment in sitting

Offer the model a blanket to put over the other shoulder and wrap it obliquely across both aspects of the trunk to cross under the axilla of the arm to be massaged. The two ends can often be tucked in to secure the blanket. Check that the blanket does not hang on the floor as the model sits down. Provide a 76 cm (30 in) or higher table with a top about the size of a standard pillow. Place a pillow on the table. Strap it if it is likely to slip, and cover with a cotton sheet. Place the model's arm on the pillow so that it rests in a comfortable degree of shoulder abduction and elbow flexion, and so that the pronated finger tips just reach the front of the table (Fig. 4.1(a)).

You should stand in walk standing at the end of the table, your outer leg forward so that you face along the forearm.

For a treatment in lying

Prepare a couch as for treatment of the lower limb, and ask the model to lie down using only two head pillows. Place a pillow alongside the trunk so that the arm can rest on it in a degree of slight abduction and flexion of the shoulder. Ensure the pronated hand is fully supported on the pillow; if not, pull the pillow down slightly leaving the shoulder area unsupported.

You should stand in walk standing just beyond the model/patient's finger tips with your outer leg forward.

To elevate the arm

Position the model in lying as for an arm treatment, but use additional pillows to ensure that each more distal joint is higher than its proximal neighbour, i.e. elbow higher than shoulder, wrist higher than elbow.

It may be necessary either to lower an adjustable couch or for you to stand on a platform in order to reach. In the absence of either facility it is possible to work backwards, but do remember to keep looking round at the model's face.

Before starting work, uncover the whole limb in order to examine it. Follow the procedure described on p. 8, and especially check by observation the state of the skin for abrasions and dryness, and the posture of the joints

which may need extra support. Then palpate –
run your hand down the length of each aspect
of the limb and note temperature, tenderness
and muscle tone.

Effleurage

Effleurage to the whole limb

Effleurage to the upper limb is usually performed with one hand at a time while the other
hand controls both the stability of the limb and
the position of the hand. The grasp on the hand
should be with your own palm cupped so you
obtain a contact with only your own palmar
margins, so that a 'sticky' grasp does not arise.

Extensor aspect

Grasp the pronated hand as in Fig. 4.1(a) with
your hand nearest to the model. The working
hand – the furthest from the model – is inserted
under the little finger and proceeds up the ulnar
border of the forearm and the medial surface of
the arm, to the axilla (Fig. 4.1(b)). The second
stroke starts on the back of the fingers, and goes
up the back of the forearm and the posterior
surface of the arm to the axilla. Turn the
forearm to mid-pronation and start the third
stroke on the thumb (Fig. 4.2); continue up the
radial border of the forearm and the lateral
surface of the arm to the axilla.

Flexor aspect

As your working hand returns, grasp the
model's hand and maintain the mid-pronation.
Your former grasping hand works from the
thumb (Fig. 4.3(a)), over the lateral border of
the forearm and the lateral surface of the arm
(Fig. 4.3(b) and (c)) to the axilla. Turn the palm
into more supination and take the fifth stroke

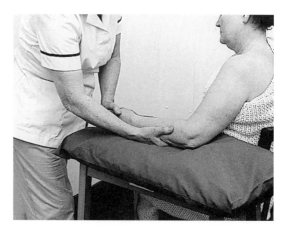

(a)

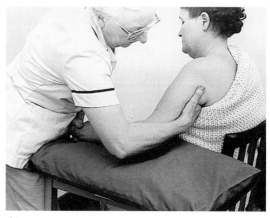

(b)

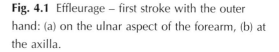

Fig. 4.1 Effleurage – first stroke with the outer
hand: (a) on the ulnar aspect of the forearm, (b) at
the axilla.

from the palmar aspect of the fingers over the
front of the forearm and the anterior surface of
the arm to the axilla. The sixth stroke goes from
under the little finger, up the ulnar border of the
forearm and the medial surface of the arm to
the axilla.

Every stroke starts with your fingers in most
contact and leading the way until you reach the
model's wrist, when your working hand, now
in full contact, should lie obliquely on the limb.

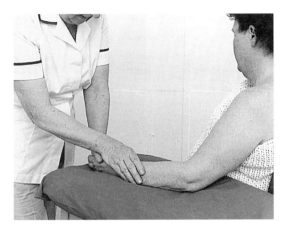

Fig. 4.2 Effleurage – third stroke with the outer hand on the forearm.

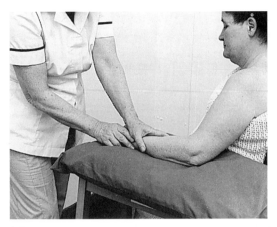

(a)

At the axilla your hand should proceed with increased depth into the area of the space by at least the length of your working fingers and pause momentarily there.

In effect these strokes have great overlap on one another, but do create a feeling of thorough cover of the part.

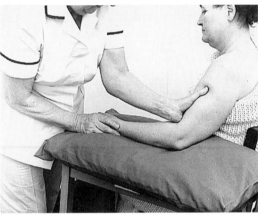

(b)

Part strokes

The shoulder is effleuraged by crossing your hands to rest one each side of the shoulder. As the strokes are made, the hands are uncrossed and turned to allow the deltoid to be effleuraged,as the fingers enter the axilla.

The arm may be effleuraged on its own, starting at the elbow and finishing at the axilla using the pattern of full length strokes described on pp. 48–49.

The forearm may be effleuraged either from the wrist, or the finger tips, to the anterior aspect of the elbow where some glands lie. Use the appropriate parts of the full length strokes described on pp. 48–49.

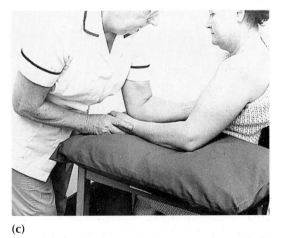

(c)

Fig. 4.3 Effleurage with the inner hand: (a) on the wrist; (b) on the arm – note the good contact; (c) at the axilla.

The hand may be effleuraged using the whole of your hand or individual structures may be treated by using your thumb or finger tips.

The interosseus spaces of the dorsum may be effleuraged using your thumbs in alternate spaces and working simultaneously (Fig. 4.4). The palm may be effleuraged using your thumbs or one or more fingers. By selecting anatomical features, such as abductor pollicis brevis and abductor digiti minimi to be treated simultaneously, your two thumbs can work together. The two flexors, and then the two opponens muscles can also be treated by your two thumbs, whereas three fingers will cover a less defined field.

The digits can be effleuraged in pairs – two with four, and three with five. The thumb can be effleuraged on its own. Balance the tip of each finger on your own middle phalanx and perform a stroke up one side with your index finger (Fig. 4.5(a)) and then up the other side with your thumb (Fig. 4.5(b)). This trick keeps the finger under treatment straight. If the fingers are a problem for this method, then grasp the tip gently with one of your index fingers and thumb and stroke up each side with the index finger and/or thumb of your other hand. It is more usual to stroke the sides of digits as the greatest drainage occurs there.

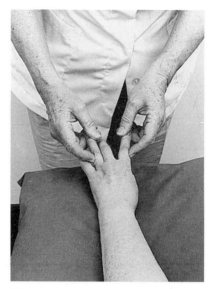

(a)

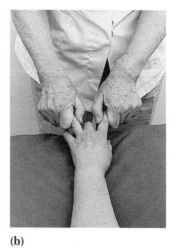

(b)

Fig. 4.5(a) Finger effleurage to the digits. (b) Thumb effleurage to the same digits.

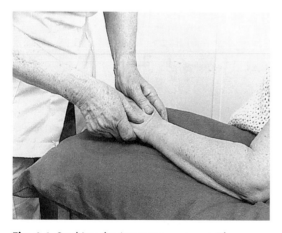

Fig. 4.4 Stroking the interosseus spaces. The same hand position is used for kneading the spaces.

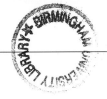

Kneading

All the kneading manipulations described are performed using the circling technique described on p. 12 (Fig. 2.4(b)). Always be aware that the size of the circle must be related to the size of the area under treatment. Ensure you are working on muscle or soft tissue and avoid deep, moving pressure over bony ridges and prominences. The pressure on all the manipulations should be inwards towards the centre of the arm and with upward pressure so that you can envisage assisting venous blood and lymph flow from distal to proximal.

Double-handed alternate kneading

Double-handed alternate kneading of the upper limb is usually performed straight down the length of the limb, from the shoulder to the finger tips, rather than sectionally as for the longer and more muscular lower limb. In consequence, the sequence of work involves careful manoeuvring of your hands so as to turn the 'corners' and to maintain full hand contact. Thus the hands start cupped over the shoulder and deltoid, encircle the upper arm to work on triceps and biceps, and turn at the elbow to lie obliquely on the flexor and extensor aspects of the forearm and hand.

Start by reaching hard with your arms and your shoulder girdle so that your hands can rest over the shoulder joint, with your finger tips touching on top (Fig. 4.6(a)). Your elbows should be bent to allow your forearms to be parallel to the table top. Knead with alternate hand circles and inward pressure, slowly pivoting on your finger tips so that the heels of your hands move to rest over mid-line of deltoid – about six to eight circles with each hand (Fig. 4.6(b)).

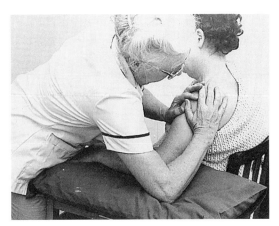

(a)

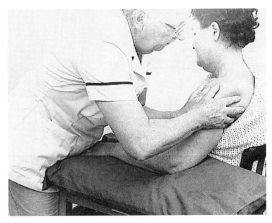

(b)

Fig. 4.6 Kneading deltoid: (a) Start; (b) finishing positions for hands.

Next, work down on deltoid in very small stages keeping your hands parallel and your thumbs touching, until your fingers can slip into the axilla. Your hands should now rest with the mid-line of each hand on the vertical mid-line of the bellies of triceps and biceps. Your fingers may overlap over the medial border of the humerus (Fig. 4.7).

The kneading should now be less of a compressive manipulation, and have an element of

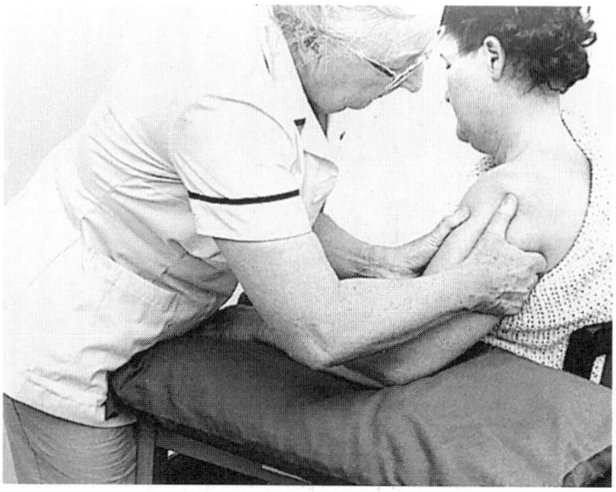

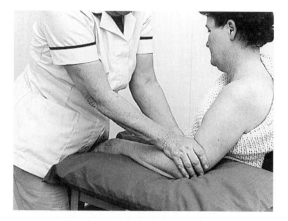

Fig. 4.7 Kneading biceps and triceps.

Fig. 4.8 Kneading – turning the elbow.

squeeze with each hand, but, as you must keep your thumbs lying vertically and close together on each side of the lateral border of the humerus, the squeeze is effected by the thumb and thenar eminence on one side and the palm and fingers on the other side of each muscle.

Proceed down the upper arm, manoeuvring your hands gradually in the lower third so that the hand on triceps comes more to the front of the elbow, and that on biceps lies more to the back of the elbow (Fig. 4.8). Let your front hand perform stationary work, while your rear hand works and slides gradually under the medial side of the elbow and on to the flexor aspect of the forearm, followed by the other hand on to the extensor aspect of the forearm.

The kneading on the forearm is done by letting your hand on the flexors lie across the limb and in advance of your hand on the extensors, which should lie obliquely but with a more vertical alignment (Fig. 4.9). In this way both your hands can maintain full contact, and the hand on the flexors can slightly lift the model's forearm to allow your hands to move down

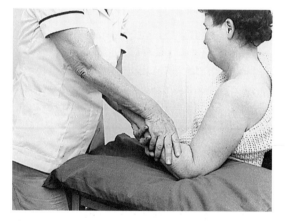

Fig. 4.9 Kneading on the forearm – note the lifted position to facilitate the manipulation and the practitioner's hands both in contact yet in different dispositions.

more easily. Your hands will catch up with each other to work at the same level on the model's palm (Fig. 4.10), continuing until his or her fingers lie in the middle of your palm. Any part of this sequence may be used to treat any specific muscle(s).

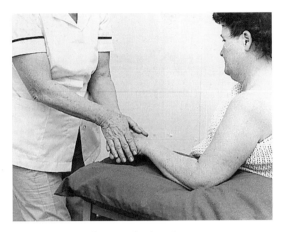

Fig. 4.10 Kneading on the hand.

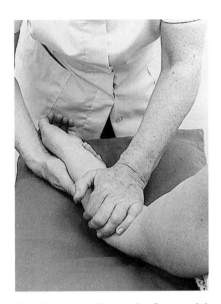

Fig. 4.11 Palmar kneading to the flexors of the forearm.

Single-handed kneading

On deltoid

The whole of one of your hands may be used to knead the deltoid muscle. The outer hand is the easier to use, and your inner hand should support the model's arm just below the axilla and on the medial side, in order to give counterpressure and stabilise the area.

On triceps

Triceps is kneaded with your outer hand, and counterpressure with your other hand is given initially halfway down, then at the distal part of the biceps.

On biceps

Biceps is kneaded with your inner hand, with counterpressure with your other hand over the mid-point and then the distal part of triceps.

On the extensors of the forearm

The forearm extensors are kneaded with your outer hand starting above the elbow flexure (remember some of the muscles take origin above the flexure), and working down to the wrist, eventually using your palm only. Support is given with your inner hand over the wrist to prevent it moving and also to raise the forearm if necessary.

The flexors of the forearm

The forearm flexors are treated in a similar way, using your inner hand starting in the elbow flexure with the whole hand, and gradually using only your palm as you work down to the wrist (Fig. 4.11). The wrist is supported with your outer hand.

The hand

The dorsum of the hand is kneaded using the palm of your outer hand, while supporting the model's palm with the palm of your inner hand. Try to cup this palm so that sticky contact of the middles of two palms is avoided. The supporting hand should be placed across the supported palm so that your fingers lie on one side, and your thumb on the other side.

Some people find it easier to learn single-handed kneading before learning to use both hands.

Finger kneading

The palm of the hand is more usually kneaded with either all or most of the fingers using flat fingers to fit over the muscle areas. Your outer hand supports the supinated hand on the dorsum to allow the middle of the palm, then the hypothenar area, to be treated. Your hands change roles and the hypothenar eminence is grasped to allow your outer hand to work on the thenar area. Finger pad kneading can be performed on each small area and eventually on individual intrinsic muscles working from proximal to distal.

Thumb kneading

Thumb kneading is more usually performed on the flatter or smaller muscle groups of the upper limb.

The flexors and extensors of the forearm

The flexors and extensors of the forearm are treated similarly. Hold the forearm a little elevated from the pillow so that your fingers can lie on the opposite aspect. Obtain maximum contact with the length of your thumbs by keeping your forearms low and parallel with the model's forearm. Then, perform maximum size circles without skin drag, and be aware that the appearance of a wrinkle above the working thumb means that your range is enough, and skin drag will follow if you con-

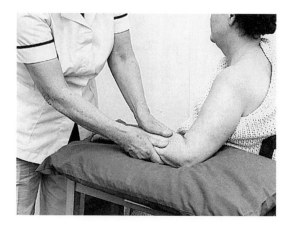

Fig. 4.12 Thumb kneading to the extensors of the forearm. Note the skin wrinkle at the tip of the right thumb.

tinue with pressure (Fig. 4.12). Ensure your thumbs pass one another 'off-contact' just sufficiently to allow the relaxed thumb to pass adjacent to the lateral border of the working thumb. **Do not press most with the metacarpo-phalangeal joint** of your thumb – avoid this by maintaining **very slight** flexion at this joint, thus avoiding hyperextension of your thumb. The manipulation is deeper on the muscle bellies, and much lighter on the distal half to third of the forearm. The extensors are treated from above the elbow flexure anterior to the lateral epicondyle, and the flexors from below the elbow flexure and distal to the medial epicondyle.

The interosseus spaces

The interosseus spaces are kneaded on the dorsal aspect using the sides of your thumbs. The manipulation has a long, narrow oval shape and is usually performed in alternate spaces, i.e. 1 and 3, 2 and 4. Support the palm with your fingers and work from proximal to distal, having determined the length of the space by stroking up it (Fig. 4.4).

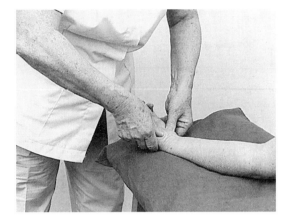

Fig. 4.13 Simultaneous thumb kneading to the abductor pollicis brevis and abductor digiti minimi.

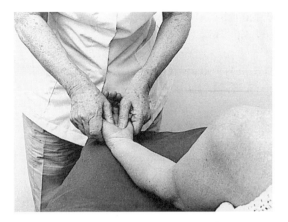

Fig. 4.14 Alternate thumb kneading to the centre of the palm.

The thenar and hypothenar eminences are thumb kneaded by supinating the hand and:

either using both your thumbs alternately on each eminence in turn *or* using one thumb on each eminence and selecting the appropriate pairs of small muscles. The abductor digiti minimi and abductor brevis pollicis are kneaded simultaneously and together, the flexor brevis pollicis (Fig. 4.13) and flexor digiti minimi are treated together and simultaneously, then the centre of the palm (adductor pollicis) is kneaded with both thumbs alternately (Fig. 4.14). This sequence prevents the wrist from being rocked sideways as the manipulations are performed. Use your thumb pads or tips for these manipulations.

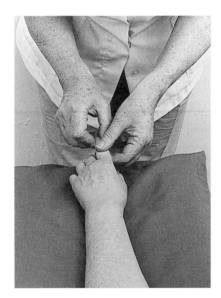

Fig. 4.15 Kneading one digit at once.

The fingers

The fingers can be kneaded in two ways. Turn the hand into pronation and:

either hold the tip of one finger in one hand, and use the thumb pad and pad of the index finger of the other hand, one on the front and one on the back of the finger near the cleft, to knead both aspects at once or first one aspect, then the other (Fig. 4.15)

or hold the proximal phalanx of two alternate fingers cupped on the middle phalanx of your index finger. Your thumb pad should be on the dorsum of the same area of the same finger. Now, squeeze knead by working first with your thumb then with your cupped finger while counterpressing with the opposite component, and proceed from proximal to distal working with both your hands simultaneously (Fig. 4.16). The other two fingers are treated in the same way, then the thumb is treated alone, using one hand while your other hand stabilises the model's hand.

Picking up

Picking up on the upper limb muscles is usually performed with one hand at once, and from proximal to distal. The operator's outer hand works on deltoid, triceps and brachioradialis, and the inner hand on the biceps brachii and the forearm flexors. The free hand stabilises the limb adjacent to the working hand. Progress should be in small stages of about 1–2 cm ($^1/_2$ in–$^3/_4$ in) at a time.

Deltoid

Deltoid is picked up using your outer hand with your inner hand stabilising on the medial side of the arm near the elbow. Use a 'C' formation

of the hand (see Fig. 2.16) and find the bony margins of the spine of the scapula, the acromion process and anterior border of the clavicle. Now slip down on to the deltoid and totally off the bone. Keep your palm in contact with deltoid all the time so that you compress the whole muscle but pick up rather less of it. Your forearm should be parallel with the model's forearm and remain so as you work. The 'pick up' is performed by extending your wrist after you have grasped the muscle and you should neither pivot on your thumb and finger tips, nor lever on the heel of your hand (Fig. 4.17). A vulnerable bony area is the lateral border of the bicipital groove and your thumb should always lie lateral to it and not on it. As the muscle narrows, you narrow the 'C' shape of your hand to almost a 'V' shape.

Triceps

Triceps is treated by sliding your hand from the tendon of deltoid to the back of the arm near the axilla, so that you encompass the triceps muscle belly (Fig. 4.18). Your finger tips should

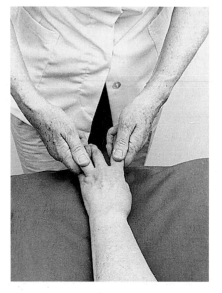

Fig. 4.16 Kneading two digits at once.

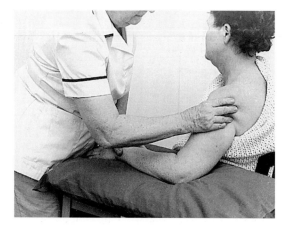

Fig. 4.17 Picking up to deltoid – note the 'C' shape of the hand.

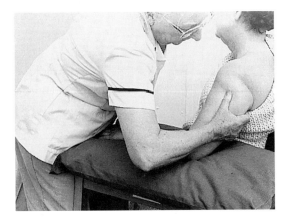

Fig. 4.18 Picking up to triceps – note the practitioner's forearm is behind the model's arm and the hand is 'C' shaped.

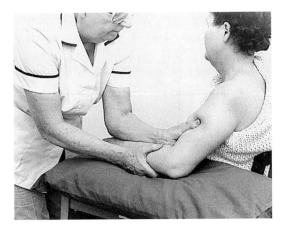

Fig. 4.19 Picking up to biceps – note the practitioner's forearm is parallel with that of the model.

lie posterior to the medial border of the humerus, and the length of your thumb should be posterior to the lateral border of the humerus. Again, keep the whole of your palm in contact with the muscle belly, and your forearm low and parallel with that of the model. Your stabilising hand should be on the biceps near the elbow.

Biceps

As triceps is completed, your other (stabilising) hand slides out of the way and up to the proximal part of biceps. Again, your finger tips and length of your thumb lie in front of the adjacent bony borders of the humerus, with your palm in full contact and your forearm parallel with the model's forearm (Fig. 4.19). As you work down the biceps muscle, your other hand should initially stabilise on the back of the elbow and move out of the way to the outside of the wrist which is lifted and the palm supinated, so that the working hand can continue to the tendon of insertion of biceps then slip medially to the forearm flexors.

Forearm flexors

These muscles are picked up using the 'V' formation of the hand (Fig. 2.17) with your fingers on the posteromedial aspect, and your thumb on the anterolateral aspect. Again, maintain full palmar contact and narrow the 'V' as you proceed down the forearm to the wrist.

Brachioradialis

This requires the use of your outer hand, so effect a smooth change by grasping and supporting at the wrist with the previously working hand, and sliding your outer hand up the length of brachioradialis to just above the elbow flexure (Fig. 4.20). Keep the forearm lifted to relax the muscle, and pick up using a 'V' formation until you reach the musculotendinous junction, which is two thirds of the way down the forearm. Many people continue to perform a picking up action as a squeeze on both aspects of the distal end of the forearm to preserve continuity of contact. At this point in a sequence on the arm, the forearm extensors are often

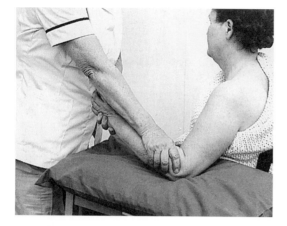

Fig. 4.20 Picking up to brachioradialis – note the 'V' shape of the hand.

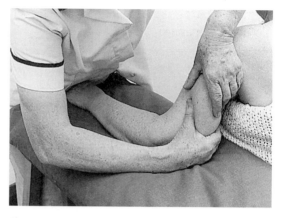

Fig. 4.21 Wringing to the triceps – note the practitioner's long reach to avoid dragging with her fingers.

thumb kneaded. Alternatively, you can return to the shoulder area to perform wringing.

Wringing

Wringing is most easily performed on the long muscles of triceps and biceps brachii. It is possible to wring a flabby or very relaxed deltoid, but the muscle is so short that it presents difficulties in performance.

Deltoid and triceps

These can be wrung by pivoting your stance and body so that you are nearer to the model and your nearest foot is between the model and the table. In both cases, your fingers should be on the back of the arm and your thumbs on the front and medial side. Ensure that these components of your hands are not lying over the adjacent bony border – the bicipital groove in the case of deltoid, and the lateral border of the humerus in the case of the triceps (Fig. 4.21). The muscles should be grasped at their most proximal end and you should work to the distal

end and perhaps return. Try to proceed in small stages so that your hands move about 2–4 cm (1 in–1½ in) at a time and move constantly.

Biceps

For biceps, you will need to move your stance slightly to the outer side of the arm support and, again, use your fingers on the medial side anterior to the medial border of the humerus, and your thumbs on the lateral side anterior to the lateral border of the humerus. Again work from most proximal to the distal part of the muscle and perhaps return, and work in small stages similar to the triceps.

Be very careful in wringing these muscles not to drag on the skin, and to keep your hand changes of direction very smooth. Dry hands are a great help in ensuring smooth, non-dragging work.

Brachioradialis

The belly of brachioradialis may be wrung using your thumb pads and the pads of your index, middle and sometimes ring fingers. The model's forearm should be fully supported in mid-pronation and supination.

Hand muscles

Tiny wringing manipulations done with the tips of your index fingers and sides of your thumb tips can be performed on the intrinsic muscles of the thenar and hypothenar eminences. The two abductor and two flexor muscles are more easily treated in this way.

Muscle shaking

Deltoid

The shorter deltoid muscle can be shaken using your outer hand. Take care not to bounce on the bicipital groove with your thumb.

Triceps

Triceps is shaken, again, using your outer hand and proceeding from near the axilla to the elbow (Fig. 4.22).

Biceps

Biceps is shaken using your inner hand, proceeding from near the axilla to the musculo-tendinous junction.

Brachioradialis

In the forearm, a bulky brachioradialis may be shaken using the thumb pad and the lateral side of the flexed phalanges of the index finger of your inner or outer hands.

The hand

In the hand you may be able to shake the bulk of both the hypothenar and thenar eminences

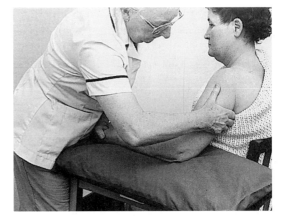

Fig. 4.22 Muscle shaking – note the loose grasp.

and, in some subjects, to select and shake the abductor brevis pollicis and abductor digiti minimi using the tips of your thumb and index finger.

Muscle rolling

Muscle rolling can be performed on each of the upper limb muscles which can be picked up, and this manipulation is often easier to perform on brachioradialis than either wringing or picking up.

Place your thumbs and fingers as though you intended to do wringing – as described above – and push the muscle belly gently first with both of your thumbs while your fingers relax but stay in contact, then pull with the distal phalanges of all your fingers while your thumbs relax but stay in contact. Proceed along the length of each muscle working down, then up, with this rocking action. Work fairly quickly and with a slight pressure inward towards mid line of the limb so that the muscle rolls from side to side.

Muscle rolling can also be performed with the thumb and finger tips on the two flexor and two abductor muscles of the thenar and hypo-thenar eminences. This manipulation can also be used to roll or 'rock' scars and adherent tissue.

Hacking and clapping

Hacking and clapping are usually performed successively to first one aspect of the upper limb, then to the other, so that the limb is moved only once.

With the model's forearm pronated, start at the posterior axilla and work down the posterior part of deltoid, triceps (reach round to the back of the arm to do so) and then on to the forearm extensors. You may need to stop the hacking at mid forearm in bony subjects, but should be able to clap on to the dorsum of the hand. Stand nearer the model for this work.

Turn the forearm to supination and lift the elbow medially, so that the limb rests comfortably on the support. Either stand on the outer side of the support, or step nearer to the model's feet, and starting at the axilla work down the front of deltoid, biceps, the forearm flexors (Fig. 4.23) and the palm of the hand, and reverse up the limb.

By working in this way you will strike the muscle fibres across their longitudinal axis. In both lines of work you should:

(1) Work in a zigzag fashion on each muscle if it is bulky or wide enough
(2) Avoid bony prominences and large tendons and jump over them:
  • At the back   the radial groove
            the lateral epicondyle
            the posterior surface of
               the distal part of the
               radius and ulna

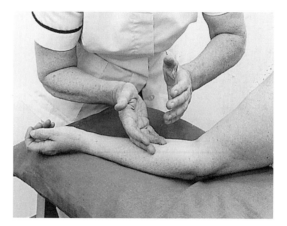

Fig. 4.23 Hacking to the forearm flexors.

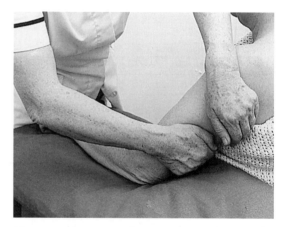

Fig. 4.24 Clapping to the upper arm.

  • At the front   the tendon of deltoid
             the bicipital groove
             the tendon of biceps
             the medial epicondyle
             the prominent carpal
               bones

Clapping is performed in a similar pattern using a more cupped hand on the more slender parts of the limb (Fig. 4.24).

Chapter 5
MASSAGE TO THE LOWER LIMB

Preparation of the model

Ask the model to remove all clothing below the waist except briefs or pants. If the model has no suitable underwear, provide him or her with either disposable pants or a loin cloth. Check that the feet are clean and not malodorous. If necessary, ask the model/patient to wash (use the excuse that a foot soak will help the treatment).

Preparation of the treatment couch

Cover the couch with an underblanket and cotton sheet, and fix them in position with straps. Provide two pillows for the model's head, and either one large pillow to go under both knees, or two small pillows to go one under each knee.

Treatment of the lower limb with the model supine

If possible the model should lie flat, but some people prefer or some patients may need, to have the elevating, head end of the couch raised so that half lying is the position used. Avoid an angle of elevation of the backrest of more than 45° so that drainage is not impeded. Cover the legs with a cotton sheet and warm covering and provide a second small cover for the upper part

of the body. If the lower limb needs elevation for the treatment of oedema, then it should be supported by pillows or by raising the end of the couch by no more than 45° (Fig. 5.1). In this case, the trunk must not be raised 45° as well. Provide additional head pillows instead of elevating the head end of the couch.

When working on an elevated lower limb, it may be necessary either to lower an adjustable couch or, if the couch is of fixed height, for you to stand on a low platform in order to reach. In the absence of either of these facilities, it is possible to turn round and face the model's feet and work backwards, but do remember to keep looking round at the model's face (Fig. 5.2).

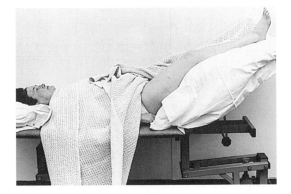

Fig. 5.1 The lower limb elevated.

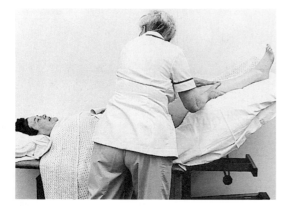

Fig. 5.2 The lower limb treated by working backwards. Note the practitioner is observing the model's face.

Treatment of the lower limb with the model prone

(To gain access to the posterior aspect of the lower limb.)

The model lies prone, with head and abdomen supported as for back massage (p. 78). Place one pillow under both ankles to allow a little flexion at both knees, and sufficient pillows under the calf of the limb to be treated so that the knee is flexed no more than 45° (Fig. 11.4). Ensure that the ankle is supported in some plantarflexion. This position is suitable for treatment of the hamstrings and/or the calf. If insufficient pillows are available, the model's ankle can rest on your shoulder, but arrange yourself carefully so that if possible you can half sit (perch) on the edge of the couch as the calf can feel very heavy by the end of the treatment and more so if you stand to work and support the limb.

Before starting work always uncover the whole limb in order to examine it. Follow the procedure described on p. 8 and especially check by observation the state of the skin for:

- Dryness
- Callosities
- Abrasions
- The presence of any varicose vessels
- The posture of the joints which may need extra supports

Then palpate – run your hand down the length of each aspect of the limb – and note:

- Temperature
- Tenderness
- Muscle tone

Treatment of the whole lower limb with the model supine

Effleurage

Effleurage to the whole limb

Stand with your rear foot distal to the model's foot, and your forward foot level with the model's calf. Both hands usually work together: your nearside hand on the sole of the foot and more medial aspect of the limb, and your more lateral hand on the dorsum of the foot and the more lateral aspect of the limb.

There are two methods of working on the foot:

(1) Each hand starts with the fingers over the toes (Fig. 5.3(a)); that on the dorsum traverses to the anterolateral side of the ankle slightly in front of that on the plantar aspect, which passes under the instep to the anteromedial side of the ankle.

(2) The alternative method of working on the foot is only different for the hand on the dorsum. For each stroke, this hand starts with the whole hand on the dorsum of the foot, the fingers over the toes and palm over the tarsus. The heel of this hand is

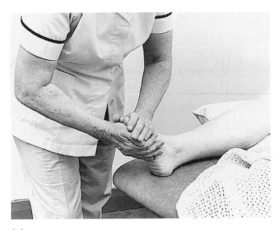

(a)

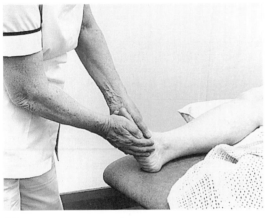

(b)

Fig. 5.3 Optional starting positions (a, b) of the hands on the foot, for effleurage to the lower limb.

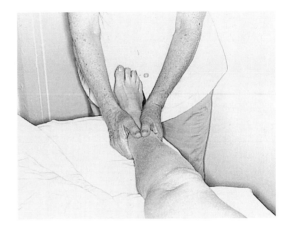

Fig. 5.4 Effleurage continues at the ankle. Note the hands moulding to the part.

near to the lateral malleolus. The stroke with this hand is initiated by pivoting it with some depth on the dorsum of the foot, so that your fingers turn to lie on the outer side of the foot and then proceed as described above (Fig. 5.3(b)). This method is useful where there is a painful ankle joint or foot as the counterpressures of the hands prevent unwanted ankle plantar-flexion which can be inadvertently caused by method 1.

Whichever method you have used you must now abduct and extend your thumbs so that your hands span first the sides (Fig. 5.4), then the front of the ankle and proceed up the front of the leg (Fig. 5.5) over the knee and thigh to the femoral triangle where you should increase your pressure and pause briefly. Throughout this part of the stroke your hands fit together (Fig. 5.6) with the thumb of your outer hand lying alongside the index finger of your inner hand. For each successive stroke your hands should fit together in this way as they come round to the front of the thigh and continue to the femoral triangle, where overpressure is given with a slight pause. The next stroke starts in the same way, but your fingers pass behind the malleoli so that your hands can continue up the medial and lateral aspects of the limb (Fig. 5.7). Your outer hand should, again, be slightly in advance of your medial hand and both move more anteriorly at the junction of the upper and middle third of the thigh so that they encompass the femoral triangle.

The third stroke starts like the second stroke, but at the malleoli your fingers pass the tendocalcaneous and proceed up the posterior aspect of the limb (Fig. 5.8) with your outer

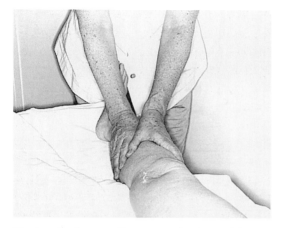

Fig. 5.5 Stroke 1 – effleurage to the front of the calf.

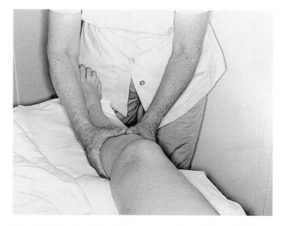

Fig. 5.7 Stroke 2 – effleurage to the sides of the calf continues up the sides of the thigh.

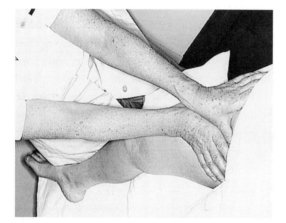

Fig. 5.6 The finish of an effleurage stroke at the femoral triangle.

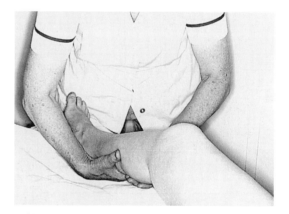

Fig. 5.8 Stroke 3 – effleurage to the back of the calf continues up the back of the thigh.

hand slightly in front of your inner hand. You will have to extend your back and lift the model's limb very slightly to proceed under the thigh from the back of the knee. At the upper third of the thigh, your hands circumnavigate to the front to finish at the femoral triangle. Pressure has to be varied to allow for the smaller ankle, bulky muscular calf, more bony knee and bulky muscular thigh. This can be best controlled by adjusting your foot positions and

ensuring your arms start to 'reach' before your body moves. You should feel your shoulder girdle protracting to assist the reaching process. At no time should you bend either your hips or your back.

Part strokes of effleurage

The thigh can be effleuraged alone if the patterns of strokes previously described start at the knee and proceed to the femoral triangle. The posterior stroke is started by sliding the hands from each side to underneath the knee.

The knee is effleuraged by crossing your hands above the patella (Fig. 5.9(a)), drawing them backwards on each side of it until the heels of your hands meet below the patella, then turning your hands to allow your fingers to pass behind the knee over the popliteal fossa (Fig. 5.9(b)).

The leg is effleuraged from foot or ankle to the popliteal fossa, following the lines of work for the whole lower limb.

The foot is effleuraged by starting in one of the two described ways and finishing at the ankle.

The interosseus spaces are effleuraged using the sides of your thumbs, meantime supporting the plantar aspect of the foot with your fingers (Fig. 5.10).

The toes. The big toe is dealt with on its own. The tip is supported on the tip of your middle finger, and your thumb and index finger stroke one up each side (Fig. 5.11). As the lateral four toes are so small, you may find you have to stroke the sides of each toe separately, balancing the tip of each toe on your middle finger and stroking up the toe on one side with your thumb and then on the other side with your index finger.

Take care to follow the basic rules for effleurage, especially ensuring you do not give maximum pressure with the leading edge of your hands.

To continue working on the thigh, cover the leg and foot with part of the covering.

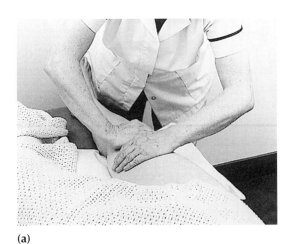

(a)

(b)

Fig. 5.9 Effleurage to the knee: (a) start, (b) finish.

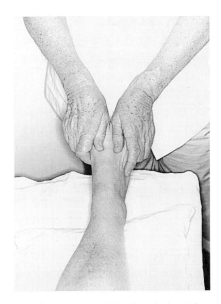

Fig. 5.10 The position of the hands for either an effleurage stroke or kneading to the interosseus spaces of the foot.

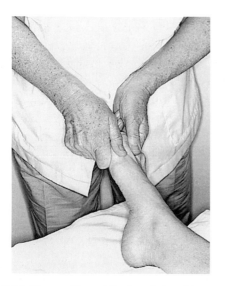

Fig. 5.11 The position of the hands for either an effleurage stroke or kneading to the toes.

Kneading

All the kneading manipulations on the lower limb are performed using the circling technique described on p. 13 (Fig. 2.4(b)) with modifications for the size of the area under treatment. Ensure you are working on muscle or soft tissue and avoid deep, moving pressure over bony ridges and prominences. The pressure of all the manipulations should be inwards to the centre of the limb with an upward inclination so that you can envisage assisting venous blood and lymph flow from distal to proximal.

Kneading to the thigh

The thigh is usually treated with double-handed, alternate kneading dealing with the medial and lateral aspects together, and the anterior and posterior aspects together. Consider the anatomy: the hamstrings extend from the ischial tuberosity to the tibia, and the rectus femoris extends from the ilium to the patella. Two groups extend the whole length of

the thigh so, except on the medial aspect, the manipulations start as high as your hands can be placed and continue to the knee.

The adductor group occupies most of the upper medial half of the thigh, and vastus medialis the lower half. On the lateral side is vastus lateralis, covered by the strong fascia lata and extending most of the length of that side. Thus there is a long length on the lateral side, and less than half that length on the medial aspect. The adductors are rarely treated in a routine practice. Specific manipulations may be used in groin strains of adductor longus tendon, but on the whole the upper medial aspect of the thigh is not massaged as the cutaneous nerve supply of the area is shared by the external genitalia.

Stand in walk standing at the level of the lower calf with your outer foot forward. For the lateral and medial lines of work, the lateral hand initiates the kneading at half tempo and works down the thigh until it is opposite the medial hand, which is resting ready on the middle of the medial aspect. This hand now works alternately with the other hand to continue to the knee (Fig. 5.12(a)). For the anterior and posterior lines of work, the anterior and posterior muscles are kneaded:

either by remaining in the same posture as for the lateral/medial aspects and inserting your nearer (medial) hand under the thigh from the inside to work on the hamstrings, while your outer hand works on the anterior aspect (Fig. 5.12(b))

or by turning your body more to face across the thigh, you then insert your hand nearest to the model's hip (outer hand) under the thigh from the outside and the further, formerly medial hand works on the anterior aspect (Fig. 5.12(c)).

In order to work deeply on these great muscle masses you must lean forward with a straight

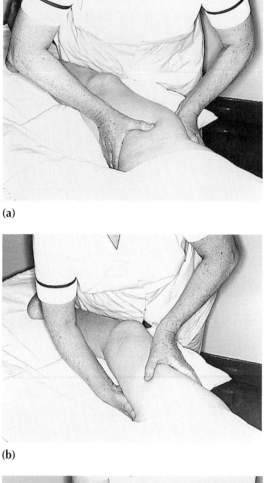

(a)

(b)

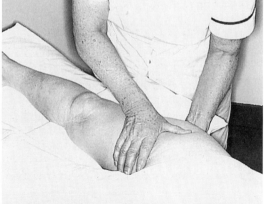

(c)

Fig. 5.12 Kneading – the thigh: (a) medial and lateral aspects; (b) one method for the anterior and posterior aspects; (c) alternative method for the anterior or posterior aspects.

back, working always with your hands in front of the level of your shoulders. As your hands proceed down the thigh, transfer your weight from your forward to your rear foot, but your weight must also be transferred constantly from one foot to the other by pivoting your pelvis. Your weight should be more on the forward foot when kneading with the outer hand, and more on the rear foot when kneading with the inner hand.

When you work on the thigh muscles keep the anatomy constantly in mind and envisage straight lines down the length of the centres of the muscles you are working upon. Keep the middle of your hand along this line so that you do not work across two muscles or muscle groups at once, which is much harder work for you as well as less effective and less comfortable for the model.

Kneading round the knee

Whole-handed kneading round the knee should extend from just above the superior margin of the synovial membrane to a hand width below the flexure of the knee so that you encompass all the structures in the region. Start with both hands on the anterior aspect with the heels of the hands touching above the patella. Work down, letting the heels of your hands divide round the patella to avoid working over it. Let the heels of your hands meet again below the patella. Next, insert each hand from opposite sides under the lower thigh until your fingers overlap. Now work down on this aspect, covering the same level as in the previous line of work.

Thumb kneading round the patella

Use the maximum length of your thumbs and work:

either with your thumbs one on each side of the patella, i.e. starting near each other and dividing round the bone margin (Fig. 5.13(a)) *or* with both thumbs working adjacent and alternately round every aspect of the patella margin (Fig. 5.13(b)).

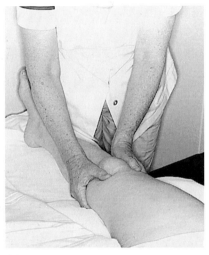

(a)

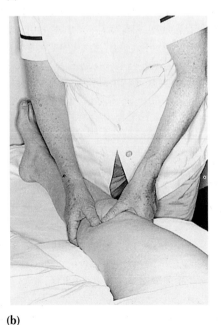

(b)

Fig. 5.13 Optional methods (a, b) of thumb kneading to the knee.

Finger kneading at the knee

Use your fingertips to work on each side of the bony areas of the knee with your thumbs resting on an adjacent area. Place your fingertips in a linear formation on first one side, then the other, of the tendons of the hamstrings at the knee so that one hand is on biceps femoris and the other on the semimembranosus and semitendonosus tendons.

If you are practising the kneading manipulations to increase your skill, continue on to the leg and foot – in which case, cover the thigh and uncover the leg and foot and continue as described below. If you are working on each area to give treatment, then complete all the manipulations for the thigh, in which case turn to pp. 71–73 for the petrissage manipulations, and to pp. 75–76 for the tapôtement manipulations for the thigh.

Kneading the calf muscles

Stand in walk standing distal to the model's feet. The lower limb may be flexed with the foot resting flat on the couch to give better access, but it is feasible to perform the double-handed kneading with the limb flat, although you should push the knee pillow higher under the thigh so that the lower edge is at the level of the knee flexure. Insert one of your hands from each side under the calf so that your fingers overlap. On the medial side, the heel of your hand must be behind the medial border of the tibia, and the heel of your hand on the lateral side must be behind the line of the fibula (Fig. 5.14).

As you knead, ensure your fingers stay overlapped. Some people actually interlock their fingers, but you may find this difficult as you work down to the narrower ankle area. Your hands should overlap more as the manipulation proceeds down the limb so that eventually one is superimposed on the other. The deeper hand

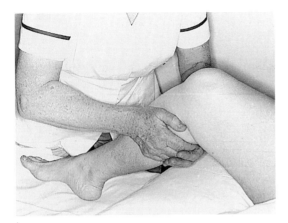

Fig. 5.14 Kneading to the calf muscles. The knee has been flexed for the photograph.

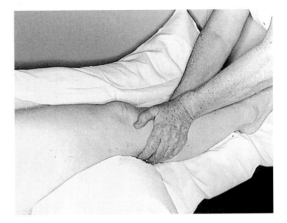

Fig. 5.15 Palmar kneading to the anterior tibial muscles.

performs the kneading, and the outer hand circles with it and reinforces if need be.

Palmar kneading to the anterior tibial muscles

Place your palm, thumb closed to it, over the upper extremities of the anterior tibial group with your fingers off-contact. Stabilise the limb with your other hand. Work down the muscle, coming more to the front of the limb as the muscle bulk diminishes, and continue on to the dorsum of the foot to the insertions of the muscles on the medial aspect of the foot, and on the toes (Fig. 5.15).

Palmar kneading on the peronei

Place the palm of your hand, thumb closed to it and fingers off-contact, on the upper limit of the peronei and work down the lateral aspect of the calf to above the lateral malleolus.

Kneading to the foot

Move the pillow to support the leg and to keep the model's heel off the couch. Place your outer hand on the dorsum of the foot, with your fingers lying laterally and your thumb below the medial malleolus (Fig. 5.16). Place your other hand on the sole of the foot, with your thenar eminence fitted into the medial longitudinal arch, fingers on the lateral side and thumb under the medial malleolus.

Work down the foot with a kneading manipulation which should also squeeze. You will find that you must always maintain some pressure with both hands all the time, or the foot will rock back and forth. Continue kneading until the toe tips rest in the middle of your palms.

Thumb kneading to the anterior tibial muscles

Medially rotate the whole limb slightly, and place both thumbs as flat as possible on the upper extremity of the bulk of the anterior tibial muscles. The remainder of your hands should rest round the calf, so that the palms are off-contact, but the fingers are supporting the limb (Fig. 5.17). Carry out a kneading manipulation so that the thumbs work throughout their length and, by bypassing one another, the

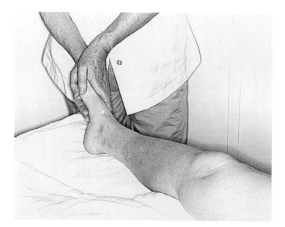

Fig. 5.16 Kneading to the foot.

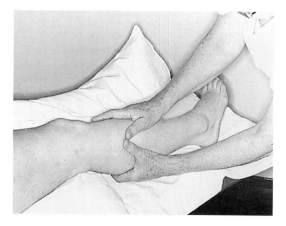

Fig. 5.18 Thumb kneading to the peroneal muscles.

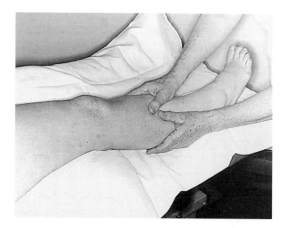

Fig. 5.17 Thumb kneading to the anterior tibial muscles (note the skin wrinkle).

thumb pads on the upper extremity of the peronei (Fig. 5.18). The remainder of your hands rest round the calf as described above. Using only the thumb pads, work down the length of the muscles and on to the tendons as they lie behind the lateral malleolus.

Thumb kneading the dorsum of the foot

Palpate the muscle belly of the extensor digitorum brevis just anterior to the lateral malleolus. Place both thumb pads over the muscle belly and, with your fingers firmly supporting the sole of the foot, work along the dorsum using an increasing amount of the length of your thumbs until you are working over the dorsum of the four medial toes.

Thumb kneading to the sole of the foot

Lean over to put your thumbs over the medial aspect of the foot, to treat abductor hallucis and the plantar aspect in mid-line (Fig. 5.19). Turn, as in Fig. 5.20, to put your thumbs over the lateral aspect of the foot, to treat abductor digiti minimi. Palpate the line of abductor hallucis muscle belly and, using your thumb pads, work from the heel to the base of the big toe

whole width of the muscle group is treated. As you work down the part, move your line of work anteriorly so that your thumbs finish on the front of the ankle and can proceed if desired over the tendons to their distal attachments on the tarsus and phalanges.

Thumb kneading the peroneal muscles

Medially rotate the whole limb and bend yourself a little sideways, so that you can place both

Double-handed, simultaneous picking up

Double-handed, simultaneous picking up may also be performed on the anterior quadriceps (see p. 19 and Fig. 2.18).

If the model lies prone, with one or two pillows under the calf to flex the knee a little, as described on pp. 61–62, the hamstrings can also be picked up as described for the vastus intermedius and rectus femoris. If the muscle bellies are very bulky, use two lines of work, one for biceps femoris and one for semimembranosus and semitendonosus. The extent of work is from just below the ischial tuberosity to the knee flexure.

Picking up on the calf

The calf muscles can also be picked up with the model either supine or in prone lying. Only the muscle bulk can be picked up, but the tendocalcaneous is usually wrung.

Stand in walk standing level with the calf. With the model supine the best access is gained by rolling the whole lower limb laterally, and working from the knee flexure to the musculotendinous junction (Fig. 5.23). If the muscle is very bulky, it is sometimes possible to work from the lateral aspect as well, in which case the lower limb should be rolled medially.

With the model in prone lying, and the foot and calf supported on one or two pillows, the calf muscles will be relaxed at the knee and ankle, and the upper two-thirds of the calf can be picked up from the knee flexure to the musculotendinous junction.

Wringing

Wringing on the thigh

Each of the thigh muscles can be treated by wringing. Your starting position, the lines of work and length of muscle treated are the same as for picking up, with the greatest effects being achieved on the anterior, medial and posterior muscle groups, in that order (Fig. 5.24). The manipulation can be difficult on the lateral aspect. Do ensure that you have lifted the muscle and are not just wringing the skin and subcutaneous tissues. The model may be supine or in prone lying for wringing the hamstrings.

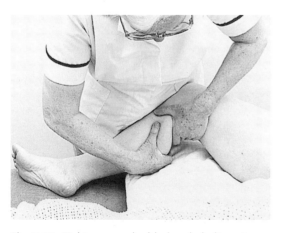

Fig. 5.23 Picking up – double-handed alternate – on the calf muscles.

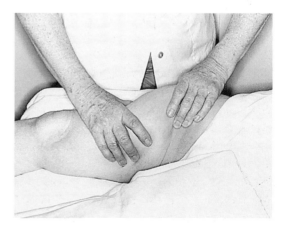

Fig. 5.24 Wringing – to the anterior thigh muscles.

Wringing on the calf

In exactly the same way as for the thigh, the calf can be treated by wringing. With the model supine, the medial half of the calf can easily be lifted and have wringing performed on it; the lateral side can be treated only with difficulty. It is very important to be careful both about 'drag' and severe compression, with your finger and thumb tips over superficial veins which may be becoming varicose. See Fig. 5.23 for the hand positions.

The tendocalcaneous can be wrung using the thumb pads and the pads of the index and middle fingers (Fig. 5.25). The basic, alternating pressures are performed on the tendon, being careful not to slip into the coulisse (the hollows between the tendon and the malleoli) on each side.

Muscle shaking

The thigh

The rectus femoris and vastus intermedius can be shaken throughout their length by placing your nearest hand on the proximal end of the muscles, and working down to the level of the upper margin of the synovial pouch

of the knee (Fig. 5.26(a)). Vastus medialis can be shaken from mid-point on the medial aspect of the thigh, working down to just above the knee.

With the model in prone lying, the hamstrings may be shaken together in the more slender subject, but in two lines of work when the muscles are bulky. For biceps femoris, your thumb should be carefully placed to the lateral margin of the muscle and your finger tips equally carefully placed on the medial margins of semimembranosus and semitendonosus.

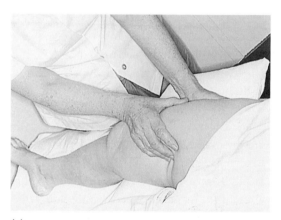

(a)

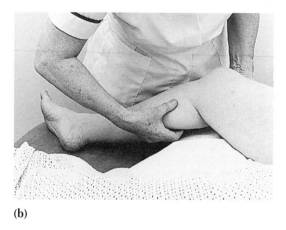

(b)

Fig. 5.26 Muscle shaking – note the fingers and thumb are in contact and the palm is off contact: (a) the thigh; (b) the calf.

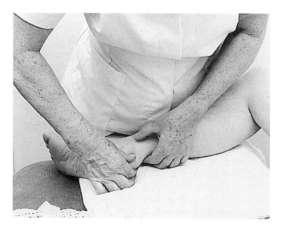

Fig. 5.25 Wringing to the tendocalcaneous.

The calf

The whole of the calf muscle bellies may be shaken, either by flexing the knee a little and rolling the lower limb laterally, then using your inside hand (Fig. 5.26(b)), or by turning the model into prone lying, supporting the lower leg and foot on pillows and, again, using your inside hand to perform the shaking manipulation.

Skin rolling and skin wringing

The knee

Skin rolling over a small range may be performed, and is useful, on the tissues round the knee (Fig. 5.27). The basic manipulation described on pp. 19–21 is adapted to be performed with the index and middle fingers on one side, and the flat thumbs on the other. It is uncomfortable when performed with too great a depth or over too great a distance. It is, however, a most useful manipulation when disease or trauma has caused the structures round the knee to thicken.

Skin wringing may also be performed for similar reasons, and may be more tolerable if small areas of skin are lifted and wrung (Fig. 5.28).

Hacking and clapping

Hacking and clapping on the lower limb are usually performed regionally. Both manipulations can be completed on the thigh before proceeding to the calf; follow the petrissage to the thigh before kneading is practised on the calf.

The lines of work should go up and down the limb, with the hands striking the muscles across their length and so across the long axis of the muscle fibres.

The thigh

For the quadriceps, start at mid-thigh on the medial side and work down vastus medialis to the knee, work to the front and continue up rectus femoris to the groin. Then move laterally to work down vastus lateralis by bending your hips and knees, after taking one pace back to get better access; then reverse along these lines (Fig. 5.29).

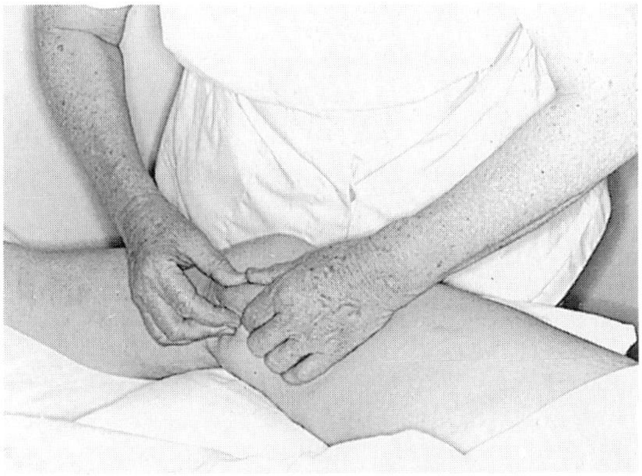

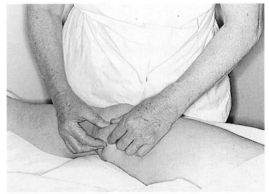

Fig. 5.27 Skin rolling round the knee using thumb and two fingers.

Fig. 5.28 Wringing the skin round the knee.

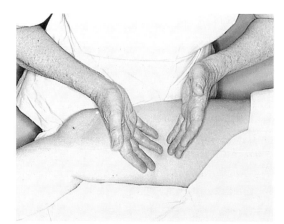

(a)

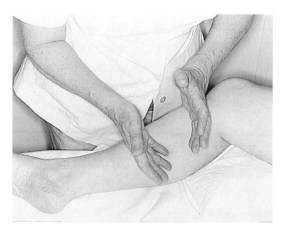

(a)

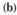

(b)

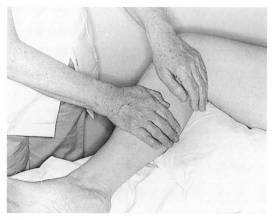

(b)

Fig. 5.29 (a) Hacking to the thigh; (b) clapping to the thigh.

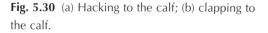

Fig. 5.30 (a) Hacking to the calf; (b) clapping to the calf.

The bony point to avoid is the adductor tubercle, and bulky muscles may need zigzag lines of hacking to effect complete cover.

The hamstrings are more accessible with the model in prone lying as for the petrissage manipulations. Medial and lateral lines of work may be necessary, working down and up semimembranosus and semitendonosus together and then biceps femoris, in each case stopping before reaching the myotendinous junctions when hacking.

The calf

The calf muscles are usually hacked and clapped by turning the whole lower limb into lateral rotation and slightly bending the knee. Work only on the muscle bulk and avoid the tendocalcaneous. Take care when hacking to avoid any varicosed vessels (Fig. 5.30).

The anterior tibial and peroneal muscles

The anterior tibial and peroneal muscles are best treated by medially rotating the whole

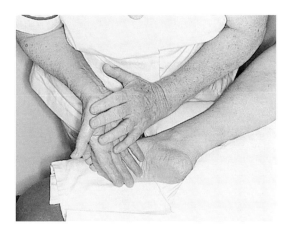

Fig. 5.31 Hacking to the foot.

The foot

Hacking on the foot is only possible on the plantar aspect of the area of the medial longitudinal arch (Fig. 5.31), and sometimes the anterior transverse arch. Both hands can be used on the former, working with the whole limb laterally rotated to give better access. One-handed hacking can be performed on the fore-foot in the anterior transverse arch, with your hand working across the line of the arch.

Clapping is best performed with one hand on the dorsal and the other on the plantar aspect of the foot, working simultaneously.

limb, more so for the peronei when you may also need to step further back with one leg, and bend your hips and knees to allow your fore-arms to be parallel with the limb. Work down to just above the level of the lateral malleolus in each case, and more lightly as the muscle bulk diminishes.

Chapter 6
MASSAGE TO THE BACK, GLUTEAL REGION AND NECK

The back and neck may be conveniently divided for treatment. The lumbar and thoracic regions are usually treated together as the 'back', but the cervical region is usually included with them for sedative treatments. The gluteal region is usually treated alone, but the lumbar region may be included with it. For treatment of the neck, the area exposed usually extends from the occiput to the lower thoracic region, so that the whole of the trapezius may be included in the treated area.

For massage to the thoracolumbar region

Preparation of the model

Ask the model to remove all clothing except briefs/pants and in the case of the female, the brassière.

Preparation of the treatment couch

Cover the couch with an underblanket and cotton sheet and fix them in position using straps. If the couch has a nose piece remove it; if not, place two pillows crossing one another at right angles at the head of the couch, so that the model's nose can rest at the crossing. Provide a small pillow to go under the abdomen and possibly one to go under the ankles. Have ready a cotton sheet to cover the body and two covers – one large one for the trunk and legs, and a small one folded to go across under the model's chest. When the model lies down, this cover should be under the breasts and, in the case of the female can be held together over the upper back when the brassière is undone and while the brassière straps are removed from the shoulders. The brassière can then be pulled out from under the model without exposing her. The outer flaps of this cover can then be used to cover the arms (Fig. 6.1). Turn the sheet and larger cover down together, so as just to expose the upper part of the gluteal cleft. Then tuck the sides of the covers under the model's hips, so that the sheet and cover are very firm and cannot be easily moved (Fig. 6.1).

Examine the area

Check by observation the state of the skin and posture; especially check that the axilla and groin are accessible. Ask the model to abduct both arms slightly so that you can insert your hands in the axilla to check if perspiration is

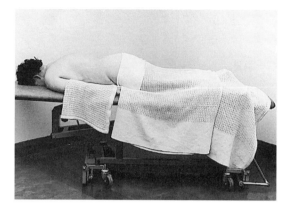

Fig. 6.1 The position of model and covers for massage to the thoracolumbar region.

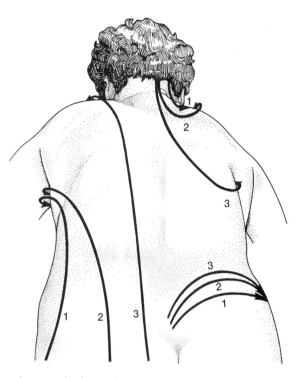

Fig. 6.2 The lines of effleurage for the lumbar, thoracolumbar and neck area.

excessive. If so, apply talcum powder. The pillow under the abdomen helps to create a triangular space to give access to the area above the groin. Slide your fingers round the sides to check that you can insert your fingers into this space (Fig. 6.3).

Effleurage to the back

The back can be divided into three overlapping areas for effleurage (Fig. 6.2). Neck effleurage is directed to the supraclavicular and axillary spaces, back effleurage to the axillary space, and lumbar effleurage to the groin. It is more usual to work bilaterally and simultaneously. Stand in walk standing at the level of the model's lower thighs and lean your trunk sideways so that you can exert equal hand pressure. Your shoulders should be parallel with the model's shoulders.

The lumbar strokes start with your hands on the middle of the lumbar region at its lowest point and finish as in Fig. 6.3, at the groin, with your fingers inserted into the space by their full length. About three strokes should be made, each with an upward curve so that the whole lumbar region is treated (Fig. 6.2).

The back strokes also start with your hands in

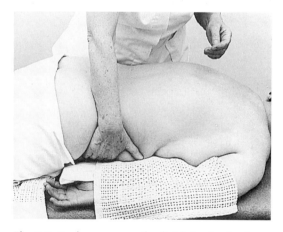

Fig. 6.3 Back massage – the finish for the lumbar strokes of effleurage.

the lumbar region. The first stroke at the sides goes to the axilla (Fig. 6.4(a) and (b)). The second stroke goes from the more central area also to the axilla (Fig. 6.5(a) and (b)). In both

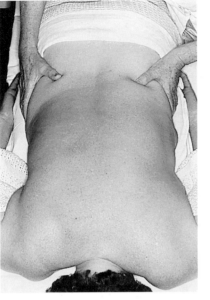

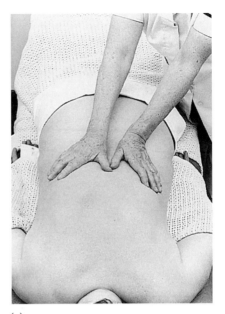

(a)   **(a)**

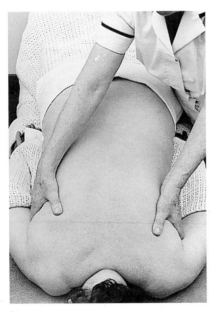

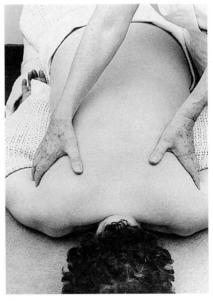

(b)   **(b)**

Fig. 6.4 Back massage: (a) the start of the most lateral stroke of effleurage; (b) the finish of the most lateral stroke of effleurage.

Fig. 6.5 Back massage: (a) the start of the two medial strokes of effleurage; (b) the finish of the second stroke of effleurage.

cases your fingers should go into the space by their full length. The third stroke proceeds up the middle of the back to the supraclavicular area, curving over the middle of the upper fibres of trapezius (Fig. 6.6).

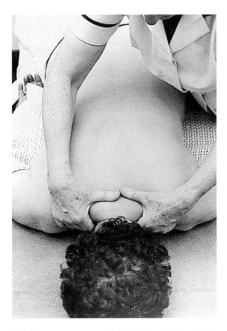

Fig. 6.6 Back massage: the finish of the third stroke of effleurage.

In all cases, ensure your hands lie obliquely on the back until the appropriate space is reached, when the stroke is terminated with the fingers leading. If you lead the strokes up the back with your finger tips your hands will be prevented from conforming to the hollows and humps of the back and may also stick and make jumpy strokes. Each stroke finishes with overpressure and a slight pause at the space.

Kneading

On the back

Kneading on the back involves keeping your hands much flatter than on the limbs, yet they

must curve to the part. The pressure is directed towards the axilla on the main part of the back in an upward and outward direction (Fig. 2.4(a)). Take care that your pressure is such that the depth treats the soft tissues. Poor direction of pressure can cause either uncomfortable compression of the trunk, or equally uncomfortable movement of the body either up and down, or from side to side on the support.

Alternate, double-handed kneading

The lines of work proceed downwards from:

(1) Just below the axilla to the outside of the buttocks
(2) Over the scapula to the buttocks
(3) Over the superior angle of the scapula to the buttocks

Work in three straight lines. A narrow back will be adequately treated with two lines of work and, obviously, a broad back may need four lines of work. Each line should overlap that adjacent by half a hand width.

Your own standing position should be walk standing, with the outer leg forward and your inner hip against the couch at about the level of the model's thighs or knees. As you work down the back, you should transfer your weight from your forward to your rear leg by gradually easing your touching thigh down the couch. In order to use your hands with even weight, lean your trunk sideways across the bed so that both elbows are nearly equally flexed and kept like that (Fig. 6.7).

As you perform the kneading, you will find that it is necessary to start with your hands slightly oblique to the long axis of the back, and to increase the obliquity as you proceed down the back so that on the lumbar region your hands may lie almost horizontally. This change in hand position is essential for maintaining full

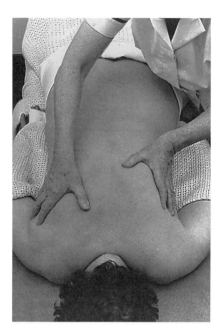

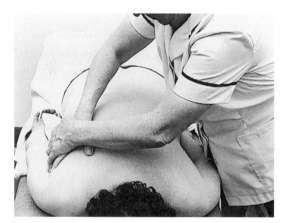

Fig. 6.8 Superimposed kneading – the far side.

Fig. 6.7 Kneading on the back. Note the obliquity of the hands and the size of the circle. The two hands are at the maximum points of their circles from each other.

hand contact (Fig. 6.7), and to allow you to work more deeply on the lumbar area. It is more usual to work with alternate hands, but more depth or more sedative work may be performed using both hands simultaneously; take care, however, not to cause the model's body to move up and down on the couch.

Do not be tempted to work at the upper back with straight elbows – this causes the whole model to move up and down on the couch.

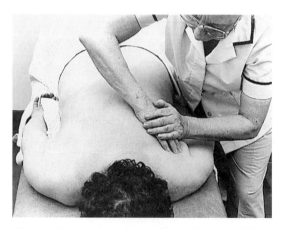

Fig. 6.9 Superimposed kneading – the near side. Note the practitioner's total change of position of feet, body and hands.

Single-handed kneading

Single-handed kneading can be performed on any area of the back. It is usual to stand in walk standing facing across the couch, and either hand may be used. Keep your other hand in firm contact, ready to change hands as you tire or as you work on another area.

Superimposed kneading

Superimposed kneading is performed for a greater depth effect than single-handed work. One hand is placed over the other as in Figs 6.8 and 6.9, and the under hand maintains the contact and pressure up and out towards the axilla, but both hands provide the depth which is transmitted from your feet.

Stand in walk standing facing across the back to treat the opposite side (Fig. 2.1), and in walk standing obliquely to the couch to treat the nearside (Fig. 2.2). On the opposite side the fingers of both your hands point outwards (Fig. 6.8) and circle clockwise. On the near side your deeper hand should point outwards re-inforced by your other hand placed in the opposite direction (Fig. 6.9), and circle counter clockwise. The lines of work are usually from:

- The axilla to the buttock
- Over the scapula to the buttock

Some people prefer always to work from proximal to distal, sliding the hands up the back to restart. Others work in a continuous line which starts under the far axilla, goes down to the far buttock, slips medially and goes up to the far scapula, slides across mid-line and reverses direction of work down to the adjacent nearside buttock and up the nearside from buttock to axilla. When this type of work is performed, difficulty may be experienced with progressing up the back without dragging on the second and fourth lines. The trick is to perform the circle and pressure, then release your pressure allowing the skin and subcutaneous tissues you have moved upwards to slide down under your hands as you start the next circle and re-apply pressure.

Thumb kneading

Stand in walk standing facing the head of the couch.

Single or double-handed, alternate thumb kneading may be performed locally to any area of the back. Your thumbs are used as flat as possible, and your finger tips should rest on the back to act as a pivot but not at a depth to perform work (Fig. 6.10).

The area most often given thumb kneading is the length of the sacrospinalis. One thumb works on each side of the spinous processes,

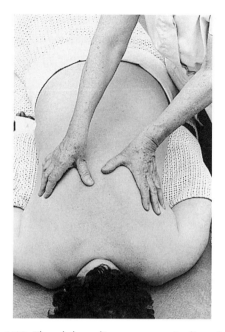

Fig. 6.10 Thumb kneading on sacrospinalis – right thumb working and left relaxing. Note their obliquity and the bulge of tissue on the outer side of the right thumb.

and the thumbs should circle round one another (not be lifted off) to move onwards. Again, use a proximal to distal sequence, starting at mid-scapular level and continuing to upper sacral level. Reach forward to start and transfer your weight backwards as in doing the alternate-handed kneading.

Finger kneading

Stand in walk standing facing the direction of work.

Finger kneading is, again, more usually performed on sacrospinalis, with the fingers of each hand on each side of the spinous processes. The finger pads are used, and greater depth is achieved if you tuck your thumbs into your palms rather than using them for support.

Localised finger pad kneading may be performed to any area such as the margins of the scapula or specific muscles in the second layer of the back, e.g. the rhomboids or the levator scapulae. In this case, always work from the margins of the muscle inwards towards its main muscle bulk (Fig. 6.11), and change direction of your stance as needed.

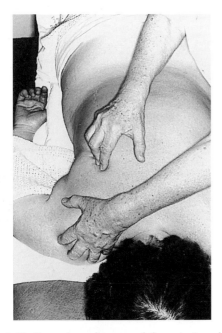

Fig. 6.11 Finger kneading round the margins of the scapula. The left hand is stabilising the scapula.

Skin rolling – back and gluteal region

Stand in walk standing facing across the couch.

The technique described on pp. 20–21 is applicable to the back, which is dealt with one side at a time (Figs 2.21–2.24). The lines of work are the same on each side except that on the side further away from you, work from mid-line to the side, and on the near side you may roll the skin from the side towards mid-line, but some people prefer to perform the manipulation by pulling from mid-line to the sides by lifting the skin with the thumbs, and thus reversing the performance (Fig. 6.12).

The lines of each rolling of the skin start from the lateral end of the spinous process of the scapula and proceed to below the axilla. The lower lines of work are horizontal from mid-line to the side. On the near side you work from the side to mid-line in straight lines, until the area below the axilla is reached when the lines spread towards the spine of the scapula. Thus on the far side you work down the back, and up the back on the nearside.

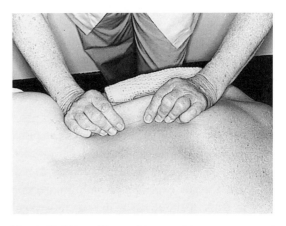

Fig. 6.12 Skin rolling – the near side.

In a similar way short lines of work can be used over the shoulders from near the acromion of the scapula to the base of the neck, working forwards from the scapular spine and from mid-line to the front and sides on each side of the neck. However, if there is considerable subcutaneous fat, the model/patient may find skin rolling in this area somewhat uncomfortable. The lines of work should be close enough together to achieve an effect on all the skin, not just on a few lines of skin.

Skin wringing

Stand in walk standing facing across the couch.

Skin wringing is not an optional manipulation to skin rolling. It is less conducive to production of a good erythema. Use it for a more mobilising effect.

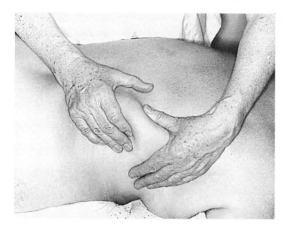

Fig. 6.13 Skin wringing.

The lines of work are as those for reinforced/superimposed kneading, i.e. down and up each side of the back. The skin is lifted up by placing your hands flat on the surface as for skin rolling, then exerting pressure with the flat fingers of one hand towards the flat thumb of the other hand (Fig. 6.13). Do not allow your hands to slide on the skin and you should obtain a roll of skin between your hands. Continuous reversal of the opposite compressing components of the hands will cause a wringing action. Do not try to work too deeply. The object is to lift and wring the superficial tissues only. Some people convert this manipulation into picking up, but the author believes that the back muscles are, on the whole, too flat to respond to such a manipulation.

Muscle rolling

Stand in walk standing facing across the couch.

Rolling of sacrospinalis is performed one side at a time. Your two thumbs form a straight line and on the far side are placed to exert pressure outwards from between the vertebral spinous process and the medial margin of the

farside sacrospinalis. All your fingertips in a straight line should be ready to exert pressure on the margin of sacrospinalis adjacent to the rib angles/lateral processes of the vertebrae. Now, alternately push outwards and with depth with your thumbs (Fig. 6.14) and then press inwards and medially with your fingertips (Fig. 6.15). Release the pressure with each set of hand components as the other set exerts pressure, and move them on to the adjacent area so that you proceed down and then up the muscle.

On the nearside of the back your fingertips. will work on the medial margin of

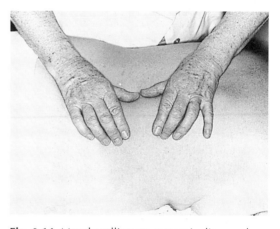

Fig. 6.14 Muscle rolling on sacrospinalis – push compression with the length of the thumbs.

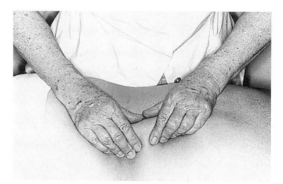

Fig. 6.15 Muscle rolling on sacrospinalis – pull compression with fingers.

sacrospinalis, and your thumb lengths on the lateral margin of the muscle. The lines can proceed from mid-scapular to the sacral region on the back.

You may be able to roll the margins of latissimus dorsi, and by careful palpation to identify and roll levator scapulae. This latter muscle is, however, more likely to need treatment with a neck condition.

Hacking and clapping

The back

Stand in walk standing facing across the couch.

Hacking and clapping on the back is done in the four lines described for kneading, i.e. two each side of mid-line, and is started under the more distant axilla.

Work down the far side, move medially and work up to below the spine of the scapula (Fig. 6.16). Jump your hands across mid-line by slightly lifting (and, in the case of hacking, pronating them more) stepping one pace backwards to do so, and continue down the medial line on the nearside of the back, then up again to the axilla.

If you wish to include the neck in the lines of work, start on the far side of the neck and work down the upper fibres of trapezius, making a little hop over the lateral part of the spine of the scapula to continue to the axilla, and on down the back. At the near side, when you reach the axilla you must turn your body towards your model's head and hop your hands over the spine of the nearside scapula to work up the nearside of the neck.

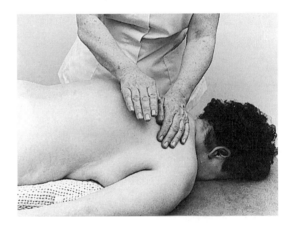

Fig. 6.17 Clapping on the back.

Clapping on the back should have a similar depth over all areas, but be lighter on the neck (Fig. 6.17). Hacking should vary in depth so that the more bony areas have lighter treatment than those that have more soft tissue bulk, where the work should be deeper.

The gluteal region

Some practitioners treat both buttocks at once, but the model/patient may suffer discomfort as bilateral work tends to separate the gluteal cleft. Much deeper work is also feasible if one side is treated at a time.

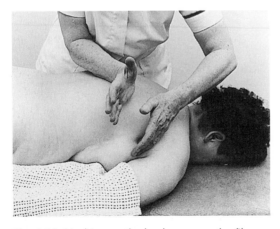

Fig. 6.16 Hacking on the back – across the fibres of latissimus dorsi.

Preparation of the model

A similar arrangement to that for the back is used, but the under-chest cover will not be needed.

To expose only one buttock, stand on the opposite side of the prone model, grasp the covers with both hands, one each at the upper and lower levels of the buttock and lift them towards you, turning the central part between your hands over as you do so. In this way, an oblong area is uncovered with the covers pleated on each side of the exposed area.

Effleurage

Three effleurage strokes are usually performed, each finishing at the groin. It is very important not to pull the buttocks apart, which is uncomfortable, and this is avoided by making every effleurage stroke curve. The first stroke is started with your hand nearest the model's feet on the middle of the buttock and your thumb on the posterior, superior, iliac spine – marked by the dimple (Fig. 6.18). Pivot your hand so

that your thumb strokes round the whole iliac crest, then adduct it to meet your palm and continue to stroke down and out until the fingers can curve under the body to above the groin (Fig. 6.19). The next two strokes curve, respectively, with an upward arc and a downward arc, from the same mid-point of the buttock to the same point above the groin. When the model is lying with a pillow under the abdomen, there is a triangular gap formed by the upper thigh, the lower abdomen and the support. This is the groin – immediately above the superior border of the femoral triangle.

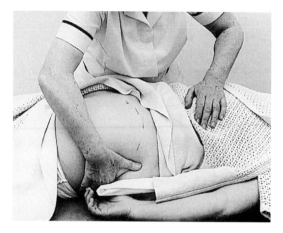

Fig. 6.19 The glutei – effleurage: the finish of all the strokes.

Kneading

As in performing effleurage, it is more usual to treat each side of the gluteal region separately. Kneading to this region is performed in walk standing facing the couch. The opposite buttock is treated.

Start by thinking of two or three lines of work which follow the lines of the main muscle fibres, which have an oblique direction from above medially to below laterally. Place one hand, usually that nearest the feet, so that it lies across the muscle fibres and over gluteus

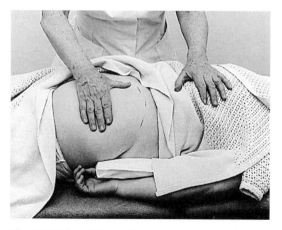

Fig. 6.18 The glutei – effleurage starting position. The thumb is on the cross marking the posterior superior iliac spine and is pivoting to stroke along the iliac crest.

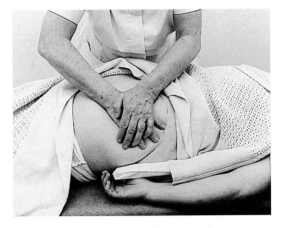

Fig. 6.20 The glutei – kneading: note the contact hand lies across the muscle fibres.

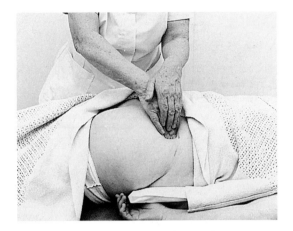

Fig. 6.21 Circular frictions to the attachments on the iliac crest.

minimus and gluteus medius (Fig. 6.20), and work down and out towards their insertions on the upper extremity of the femur. Next, move your hand, still oblique, to the origin of gluteus maximus on the iliac crest and work down and out to the fascia lata. Repeat if necessary for a third, more medial line of work.

Superimposed kneading

Superimposed kneading should be used when the muscle bulk is great, using exactly the same lines of work. The kneading manipulation, in both single-handed and superimposed work, is done in such a manner that the pressure is on to and through the glutei, and with great depth in the second and third lines of work, but on the more lateral line the pressure is directed inwards as though pulling towards yourself. The elbow kneading described on p. 17 can also be used.

Frictions

Circular frictions

Circular frictions can be performed on selected areas to achieve local, deep effects. The margin

of the iliac crest over aponeuritic structures giving rise to the muscles is an area sometimes needing attention. Use your unsupported thumb or fingers and gradually encroach inwards to the area of discomfort or disruption (Fig. 6.21).

Picking up

Work in the same oblique lines along the length of the muscle fibres as used for kneading. Stand in walk standing, using your body weight by transferring your weight forwards and backwards to exert deep pressure on the pressure phase of the picking up manipulation. Your hands will thus also have a maximum span, so that the muscles can be lifted and squeezed more easily (Fig. 6.22). The lines of work are short, and you can work up and down the muscles using single-handed, alternate picking up.

Wringing

Wringing may be feasible on some subjects. Your position and lines of work are as for picking up but the muscle bulk is passed

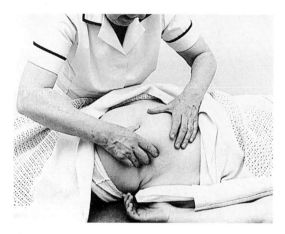

Fig. 6.22 The glutei – picking up: along the muscle fibres.

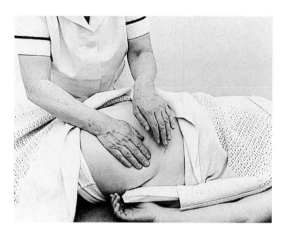

Fig. 6.24 The glutei – clapping: across the muscle fibres.

between your hands once it has been lifted by exerting pressure with all the fingers of one hand and the thumb and thenar eminence of the other hand at the same time.

Hacking and clapping

The lines of work are as for the kneading so that your hands strike at right angles to the length of the muscle fibres. Hacking the clapping (Figs 6.23 and 6.24) can both have con-

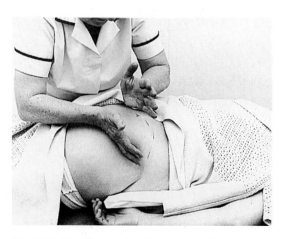

Fig. 6.23 The glutei – hacking: across the muscle fibres.

siderable depth, but very bulky tissues may need beating or pounding which can be very deep without stinging and which are less uncomfortable for the operator to perform.

For massage to the neck

There are four positions for neck massage.

Model in prone lying

A similar arrangement to that for the back is used, but the main sheet and cover are turned back to the level of the upper lumbar region (Fig. 6.1). For work in this position, stand level with the model's hips and in walk standing. Lean sideways towards the model.

Model in lying

The model lies supine with one or two head pillows. The under-covers should not be strapped down on to the couch, so that you can sit at the head of the couch and pull covers, pillows and model up the couch until the inferior angles of the model's scapulae are only just

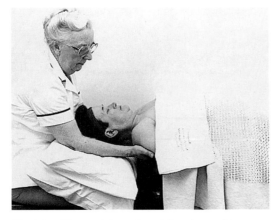

Fig. 6.25 The position of model and practitioner for treatment of the neck when it is very painful. Effleurage – neck to axilla.

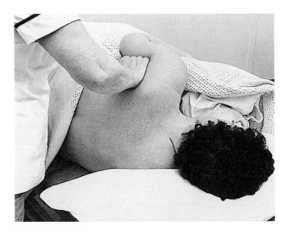

Fig. 6.26 The position of the model in side lying for treatment of one side of the neck in side lying. Effleurage – neck to axilla.

supported by the couch (Fig. 6.25). This is an excellent position in which to massage a very painful neck with much protective spasm.

Model in side lying

The position of side lying, with two head pillows and a pillow at the front of the model to support the upper arm, can be used for unilateral work. The large cover should be arranged to leave the upper side of the neck and the scapular region free to be massaged (Fig. 6.26). Stand behind the model in walk standing at about the level of his or her waist.

Model in forward lean sitting

Arrange a table against a wall and place on it a pile of pillows against which the model can lean with full support of his or her upper trunk, arms and head. Ask the model to sit in front of the table, preferably on a stool or a chair with a very low back (Fig. 6.27). Remove the top pillow and spread a large cover on top of the pillow pile and in front of the model. The model should be already undressed except for the

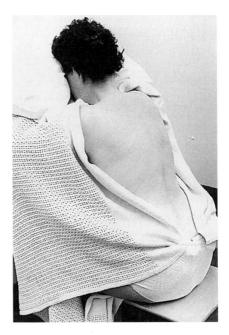

Fig. 6.27 Lean forward sitting position of the model for neck massage. Note the straight back and that the head is not flexed.

brassière in the case of a female. Ask him or her to place both arms on the pillow and cover pile, leaning forward with a straight back and neck. The upper corners of the cover are then lifted, pulled across the model's arms and tucked into the model's waistband at the centre back (Fig. 6.27). In the case of a female, the brassière can then be undone and slipped off the arms. Replace the top pillow on the pile and ask the model to lean his or her head against it. If necessary, two top pillows may be crossed as in prone lying, to accommodate the nose. Check that the forward lean is still with a straight back and neck. There should especially be no neck flexion.

Stand in walk standing behind the model, and be prepared to transfer your weight forwards and backwards, and also possibly to bend your hips and knees to gain comfortable access to the thoracic region. You may, additionally, need to take a side step to each side in turn, to gain full access or better pressure for some manipulations.

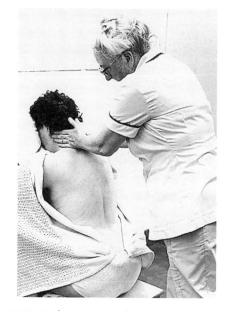

Fig. 6.28 Neck massage – the start of the more lateral stroke of neck effleurage.

Effleurage

The neck strokes are performed with the flat of the fingers starting on the sides of the neck and going to the supraclavicular glands (Fig. 6.28). A second stroke down the back of the neck, goes to the same glands, and a third stroke goes down the back and sides of the neck with more of the hand in contact, turning, over the area of the medial angle of the scapula to continue to the axilla (Figs 6.25 and 6.26).

Similar strokes to those performed on the back should also be performed when the model is in prone lying or lean-forward sitting (Fig. 6.28).

When the model is in lying or side lying the lines of work are devised to follow the above patterns, bearing in mind the need for maximum hand contact and a comfortable and effective stroke, finishing at a group of lymph glands with slight overpressure and a pause.

Kneading

The neck is a difficult area as it is so confined and may be very short in some subjects. If it is treated with the model in prone lying, then the kneading may start on the neck and proceed down to whole-handed work on the wider part of the back (Fig. 6.29). As much of your hand as possible should be used for kneading, whatever the position used for the model.

The finger pads are used on the posterior aspect from the occiput (Fig. 6.29) down to where the neck widens, and then the hands are flattened, possibly overlapped, and continue on the interscapular area. On the lateral aspect of the neck, the fronts of the two distal phalanges of all four fingers (Figs 6.30 and 6.31) are used until the swell of trapezius allows your whole hand to be in contact, using your palm at the back and your fingers at the front on the upper fibres of trapezius. A squeeze knead is now performed. Flat-handed kneading is performed on

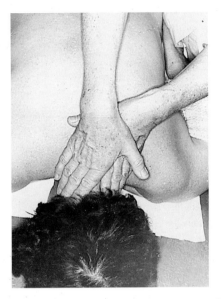

Fig. 6.29 Neck massage – kneading of the medial muscles.

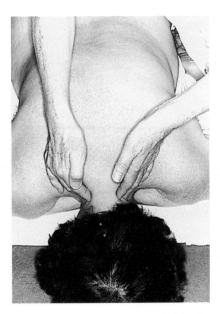

Fig. 6.31 Neck muscles – kneading of the lower lateral muscles.

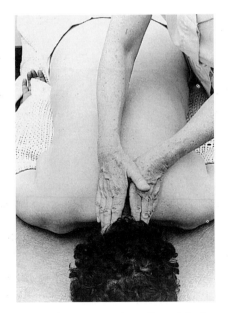

Fig. 6.30 Neck massage – kneading of the lateral muscles.

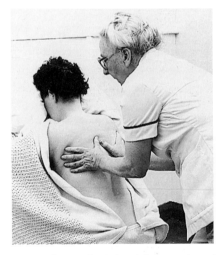

Fig. 6.32 Neck muscles – kneading continued to the middle and lower fibres of trapezius.

the upper thoracic area in a line from the inter-scapular area towards the axilla (Fig. 6.32).

When using your fingers, the pressure should always avoid contact with bone (the spinous and transverse processes of the upper cervical vertebrae) and should be upwards and inwards on the muscle bulk lying between the processes.

With careful adaptation of your hand the

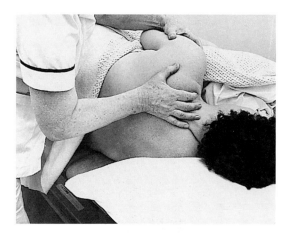

Fig. 6.33 Neck muscles – continued kneading on trapezius, with model in side lying.

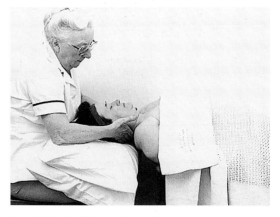

Fig. 6.34 Neck finger kneading to the posterior muscles, with model supine.

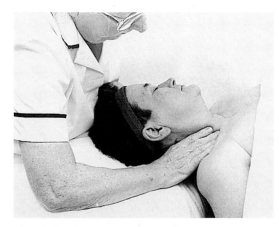

Fig. 6.35 Neck – flat finger kneading: to the scalene muscles, with model supine.

neck muscles may be treated from occipital to mid-scapular levels, and so may the upper and also middle and lower fibres of trapezius throughout their length (Figs 6.33–6.35). With the model supine, flat finger kneading can be performed on the scalene muscles.

Picking up

Place one hand round the whole posterior aspect of the neck and perform a single-handed picking up manipulation which can evolve into simultaneous work done on the lower part of the upper fibres of trapezius with one of your hands on each side of the neck. Your fingers should be over the front of the muscle and your palms and thumbs at the back. The change from one- to two-handed work must be smooth (Fig. 6.36).

Muscle rolling

The posterior column of neck muscles on each side may be rolled by placing your fingers just behind the transverse processes and your thumbs alongside the spinous processes and on the same side as your fingers (as on the sacrospinalis, p. 85). Work on each side in turn.

Sternocleidomastoid can be rolled in a similar manner (be very careful to exert sideways pressure only), if the model is in a suitable position (Fig. 6.37), but you may find it more feasible to put your index and ring finger tips one on each side of the muscle, and roll it by small supination and pronation movements.

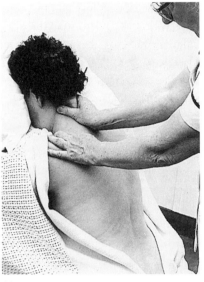

(a)

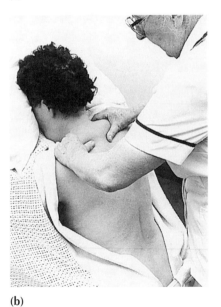

(b)

Fig. 6.36 Model in lean forward sitting: (a) a picking up type manipulation which also kneads the neck muscles; (b) continued picking up to the upper fibres of trapezius.

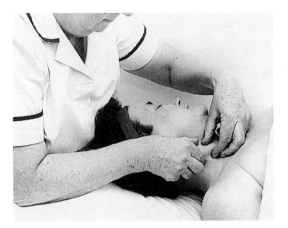

Fig. 6.37 Model supine – neck – wringing to sternocleidomastoid.

Scapula rolling

If a neck is stiff and painful, it often causes the scapula to be held in abnormal postures. When the unilateral treatment technique is used, the scapula can be 'rolled', i.e. passively taken through the movements of protraction, elevation, retraction and depression while pressure is exerted on the bone. This means that the deep, scapular muscles are intermittently compressed against the rib cage with potential effect on their blood flow.

Grasp the model's arm with your arm which is nearest to the model's head, so that the forearm is comfortably supported on your forearm. Apply pressure to the scapula with your other hand. Now, circle the scapula through all four of its movements to the maximum possible range (Fig. 6.38).

Hacking and clapping

Hacking and clapping may be performed on the neck alone, with the lines of work starting near the occiput and proceeding to the lateral part of the shoulder. Two lines may be used – one more lateral, and one more posterior on the

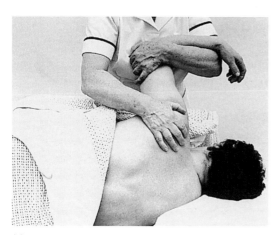

(a)

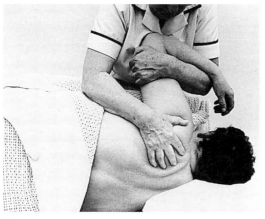

(b)

Fig. 6.38 Model in side lying – scapular rolling:
(a) protracted; (b) retracted.

neck. The more lateral line would continue on the anterosuperior part of the upper fibres of trapezius, while the more posterior line would continue on the posterior part of the same muscle fibres. Lines of work extending on to the upper thoracic region follow the lines described on p. 86.

In clapping the neck it may be necessary to work mainly with the flat fingers, and be careful not to sting. (Listen for stinging – the sound is sharp.)

Chapter 7
MASSAGE TO THE FACE

Facial massage is usually given with the model in lying, and he or she should be given a pillow under the knees, as well as pillows under the head. The practitioner will be more comfortable, and have better access, sitting at the head of the bed with the head pillows resting on his or her knee (Fig. 7.1). This position allows the practitioner's forearms to be supported for some of the manipulations, but check constantly as you work that as the model relaxes, the head does not 'sink' into the pillow causing the neck to extend and the face to tilt.

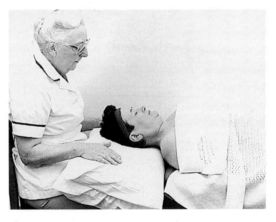

Fig. 7.1 Starting position.

Preparation of the model

Ask the model to remove outer clothing from the neck and shoulders and to remove shoulder straps. Necklaces and ear-rings should be removed as should make-up, which can become smudged. Obviously, spectacles must be removed, but discuss the removal of contact lenses with the patient. If the hair is long or likely to obstruct, it can be restrained by a headband.

Ask the model to lie down, and cover the body up to the subclavicular level if he or she so wishes. Ask the model to slide up the couch to rest his or her head on the pillows on your knee.

The manipulations for the face

Most of the manipulations are performed with the fingers or finger pads, and it is important to control the position of the rest of your hand, including the thumb, so that you do not rest on the patient's face.

The manipulations which may be used are:

(1) Effleurage
(2) Finger tip kneading
(3) Wringing
(4) Plucking
(5) Tapping
(6) Reverse finger tip hacking
(7) Vibrations to the exit foramina of the trigeminal nerve

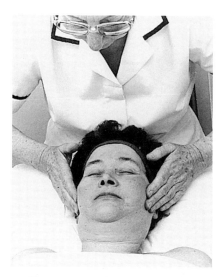

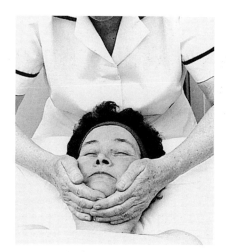

Fig. 7.3 Effleurage to the chin.

Fig. 7.2 Effleurage – the finishing position for all three strokes shown in Figs 7.3, 7.4 and 7.5.

(8) Finger kneading to the exit foramina of the trigeminal nerve
(9) Vibrations over the sinuses
(10) Occipitofrontalis stretching to obtain scalp movement
(11) Clapping to the area of platysma
(12) Stroke moulding to individual muscle(s)

Effleurage

Effleurage is directed from mid-line of the face to just below the ear (sub-auricular glands), taking care that as you stroke you do not constantly move the ear lobe.

As much of the palmar surface of the hand as possible is used to start the strokes. The finish is always with the finger pads, as the palms lift to clear the ear (Fig. 7.2).

The **first** stroke goes from under the chin – use your full hand (Fig. 7.3).

The **second** stroke starts with the fingers spread above and below the mouth – use your full hand.

The **third** stroke starts at the nose – use your finger tips to start, then your full hand (Fig.

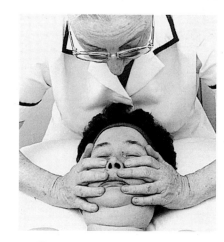

Fig. 7.4 Effleurage to the cheeks.

7.4). On a small face, the **second** and **third** strokes are often combined.

The **fourth** stroke starts in mid-line of the forehead and curves downwards – use your full hand, and repeat for a **fifth** stroke if the forehead is high (Fig. 7.5).

Kneading

The lines of work are similar to those for effleurage, proceeding from mid-line to the sub-auricular area:

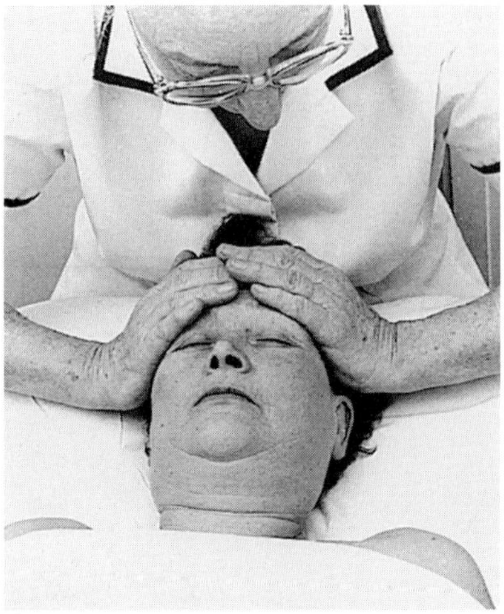

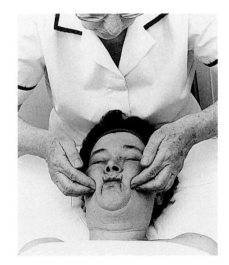

Fig. 7.5 Effleurage to the forehead.

Fig. 7.6 Kneading to the cheeks.

- The first line under the chin is done with the flat of the fingers, which are also used on the cheeks to finish the next three strokes (Fig. 7.6)
- Then the chin to ear line is started with the two distal phalanges
- Next the upper lip to ear line is started with one finger pad
- The nose to ear line is done with one or two finger pads
- On the forehead two or three lines are performed with two or three finger pads (Fig. 7.7)

All the manipulations are performed with a lifting pressure upwards and inwards so that the delicate muscles are not dragged.

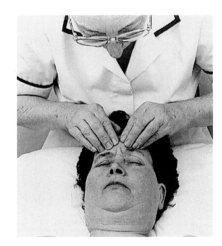

Fig. 7.7 Kneading to the forehead.

Wringing

This is a finger tip wringing performed between the finger pads of the index fingers and thumbs. It is a very small manipulation. Start at the corner of the mouth and work out to the ear, then across the chin to the other ear. Now work back to the mouth, out to the ear from the nose

on one cheek (Fig. 7.8) and across the forehead in three lines to the opposite ear, in to the nose and you are back at the start (Fig. 7.9).

Some people consider that this manipulation should be avoided when treating facial palsy, in case the muscles are overstretched, but if the depth is light and the speed is fast, there is little reason to omit the manipulation.

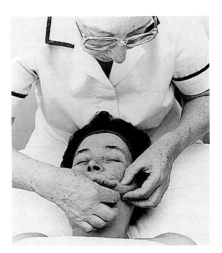

Fig. 7.8 Wringing to the cheeks.

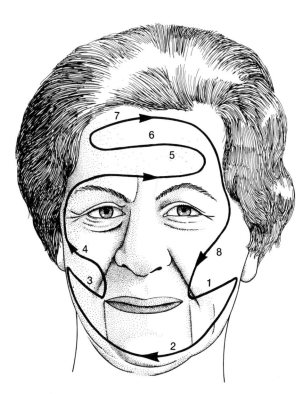

Fig. 7.9 The lines of work for wringing.

Plucking

Plucking is a stimulating manipulation performed by the tips of the thumb and index finger, in which the tissues are literally 'plucked', i.e. grasped and let go very quickly (Fig. 7.10). If the tissues were held longer you would be **pinching**. Plucking may be performed with one or both hands simultaneously, in similar work lines to kneading.

Tapping

Tapping is performed with the fingertips (Fig. 7.11). Either one, two or three finger tips are used according to the size of the area of the face being treated. If two or more fingers are used, they may tap simultaneously, or in rapid succession as in striking two or three adjacent piano keys. The tap should be firm enough to cause slight indentation of the skin at each tap. Note that the simultaneous use of two or more fingers is likely to be heavier than sequence tapping. The lines of work are those used in the effleurage. The work may be performed on both

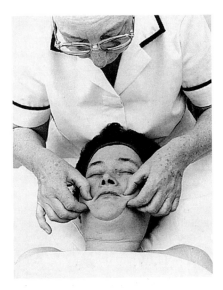

Fig. 7.10 Plucking to the cheeks.

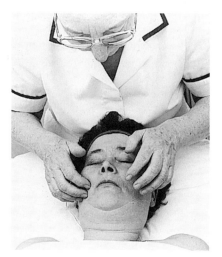

Fig. 7.11 Tapping to the cheeks.

sides of the face simultaneously, or one side of the face at a time, in which case use your other hand to stabilise the face.

Reverse fingertip hacking

Reverse fingertip hacking is performed with the palmar aspect of the medial three fingertips. The hand starts pronated and the fingers are held in slight flexion. The tissues are flicked gently with the fingertips by rapid supination of the forearm. The lines of work are those used in effleurage. The work may be performed on one side of the face or both sides simultaneously. Reverse fingertip hacking is lighter than tapping and may be used earlier when the patient is recovering from facial paralysis.

Vibrations to the exit foramina of the trigeminal nerve

Fingertip vibrations may be performed using either the index or middle fingertip over the points of exit of the ophthalmic, maxillary and

mandibular divisions of the trigeminal nerve. They emerge respectively from the supraorbital notch and the infraorbital and mental foramina. The fingertip should rest lightly over the exit and constant vibrations of a small dimension are performed until discomfort diminishes. This technique is used in the treatment of both trigeminal neuralgia and tension headaches (Fig. 7.12).

Finger kneading to the exit foramina of the trigeminal nerve

The index or middle fingertips are used to perform stationary finger kneadings over the points of exit of the ophthalmic, maxillary and mandibular divisions of the trigeminal nerve, at their respective exits through the supraorbital notch and the infraorbital and mental foramina. The finger kneadings are deeper manipulations than the vibrations described above, and are used successively with them for the same clinical circumstances (Fig. 7.12).

Vibrations over the sinuses

If the tips of your fingers and thumbs are held bunched together, and your hand is raised so that the ends of the tips rest on the skin, vibrations can be performed over a circular area (Fig. 7.13). The fingertips can be placed over the area of the frontal sinus and of the maxillary sinus, and static vibrations performed to encourage a mechanical effect on the sinuses when they are congested and perhaps blocked. The patient can be taught to perform this manipulation, and may find that the frontal sinuses are cleared best when he or she is upright and the maxillary sinuses in the side lying position. The right sinus is drained in left side lying and vice versa.

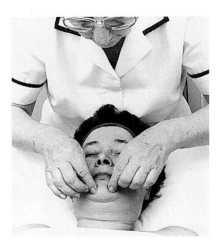

(a)

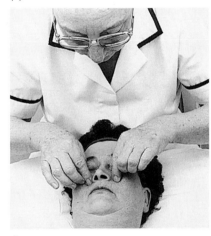

(b)

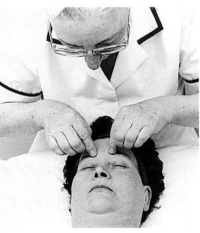

(c)

Fig. 7.12 Positions for kneadings or vibrations with one finger over the: (a) mentalis foramen; (b) infraorbital foramen; (c) supraorbital notch.

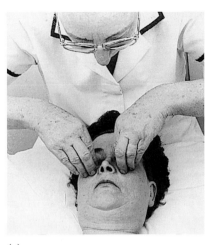

(a)

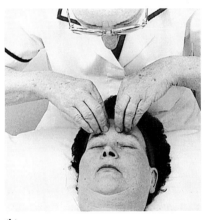

(b)

Fig. 7.13 Vibrations with all the finger tips: (a) over the maxillary sinus; (b) over the frontal sinus.

Occipitofrontalis muscle stretching

Place the palmar surface of one hand on the forehead and the palmar surface of the other hand under the occiput. Move them simultaneously so that the hand on the forehead takes the front of the scalp downwards towards the eyebrows, and the hand on the occiput takes the back of the scalp upwards (Fig. 7.14). The movement should be smooth and slow and reversed equally smoothly. The scalp will be felt to move forwards and backwards. This

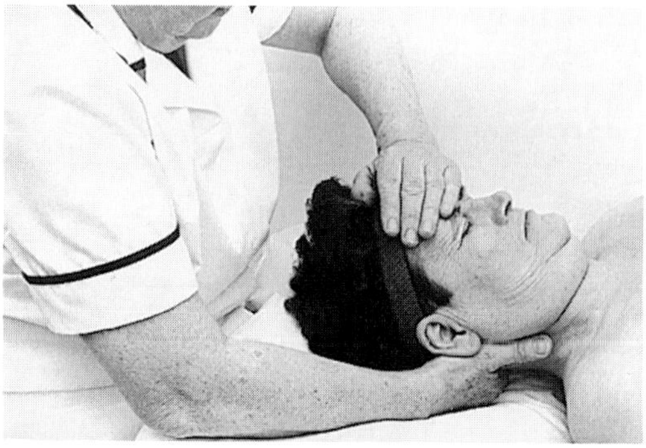

Fig. 7.14 One hand over anterior and one over the posterior belly of occipitofrontalis to rock the muscle and scalp.

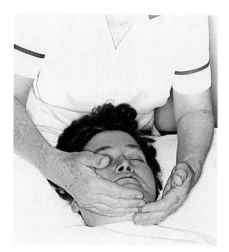

Fig. 7.15 Clapping to platysma.

stretching movement is of great use in severe headache when the two bellies of the occipitofrontalis often remain in painful spasm.

Clapping to the area of platysma

The area below the chin can be clapped using the cupped fingers (Fig. 7.15). Your hands must circle round one another in such a manner that the 'strike' is in a forward and upward direction. Be careful not to touch the front of the throat, and work at a brisk speed. The patient may learn to do this himself or herself, using the backs of the fingers.

Muscle moulding

Place your fingertips on each of the groups of muscles of facial expression in turn and mould

the muscle actions. At the same time ask the patient to attempt the muscle actions of:

* Pursing the lips
* Opening the mouth
* Producing a mirthless grin
* Smiling
* Sniffing
* Wrinkling the nose
* Scowling
* Raising the eyebrows
* Closing the eyes
* Blowing or whistling
* Expressing disgust

Chapter 8
MASSAGE TO THE ABDOMEN

The abdomen is usually massaged for one of two specific purposes. The inflated abdomen needs treatment to assist the removal of flatus and the constipated person needs treatment to stimulate the passage of faeces.

Preparation of the model

Ask the model to remove all covering of the area so that up to the lower rib case is bared as is the area to the level of the anterior superior spines. Heavy clothing on the chest and pelvis should be removed so that there is no obstruction to access by a roll of clothing. The model should wear pants or briefs and a vest or brassiere.

The model should lie supine on a treatment couch prepared with an undersheet, with pillow(s) under the knees to keep the lower limbs in a low crook position (Fig. 8.1). Small size pillows which just fit under the knees are less obstructive than full size pillows. A low raise should be applied to the head of the treatment couch; use one to two head pillows. Cover the upper chest with a small sheet or blanket folded lengthways and the lower limbs with a blanket which should be anchored on each side by being tucked under the pelvis (Fig. 8.1). If the patient can roll to each side in turn the tucking in process is facilitated. Stand on the right of the model for all procedures.

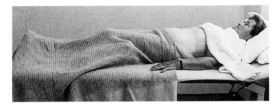

Fig. 8.1 Position for abdominal massage. Note the anchored blanket.

Palpation

The state of the abdomen must be ascertained first. Place your relaxed right hand flat over the area of the umbilicus and exert gentle pressure. This will tell you if there is any tension. Let your hand remain there as you question the model with regard to painful areas – moving to these areas in turn and gently but firmly using flat fingers to increase the depth of the palpation. If the indication is of no specific area of pain then the following sequence can be used:

(1) Run your hand over the lower ribs from left to right.
(2) Palpate below the left costal margin then the right costal margin, taking particular note of the crossing of the right lateral margin of rectus abdominus with the costal margin for the gall bladder.
(3) Now use both hands superimposed to palpate more deeply, starting in the right iliac area and paying particular attention

to McBurney's point (one third of the distance from umbilicus to the anterior superior iliac spine) and the potential content of the ascending colon. Faeces present as a firm rouleaux or as a mass. Continue to the costal margin then move to the right costal margin and palpate down the line of the descending colon to the left iliac area (Fig. 8.2). On slender subjects the depth can be moderate but on obese subjects considerable depth has to be attained before the abdominal content can be palpated.

Effleurage to the abdomen

Stand in walk standing below the level of the model's hips and lean slightly to your own right to place your right hand on the side of the upper buttock with your left hand on the left side. Start with a curved stroke going towards midline ending just above the groin. The second and third strokes each start higher at the side so that the third stroke comes from over the lower ribs (Figs 8.3 and 8.4).

Kneading to the abdominal wall

The same lines of work as in effleurage may be used and the hands should simultaneously do

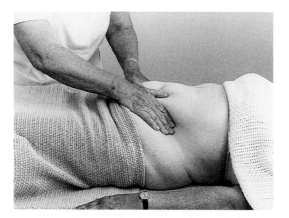

Fig. 8.3 Effleurage – the stroke is from the waist to the symphysis pubis.

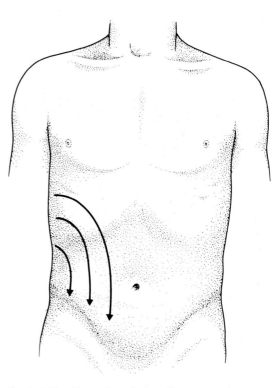

Fig. 8.4 The lines of work for effleurage and kneading.

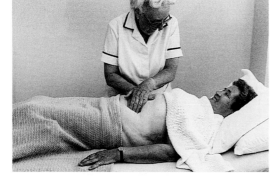

Fig. 8.2 Palpation of the abdomen.

the same thing. Do not do alternate work with your hands or the model will rock from side to side (Fig. 8.5(a) and (b)).

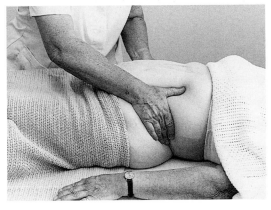

(a)

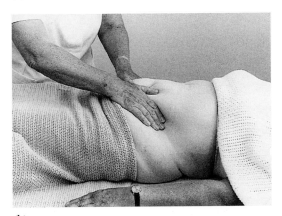

(b)

Fig. 8.5 Kneading the abdominal walk: (a) start at the waist; (b) finish over the groin.

Stroking

Stand in walk standing facing across the model and level with the abdomen. Stroking may be done across the abdomen from left to right and should be in a pattern starting from above and working down so that each stroke overlaps. Alternate hands can be used (Fig. 8.6(a)).

Alternatively, on a very tense abdomen use your right hand and execute a circular stroke

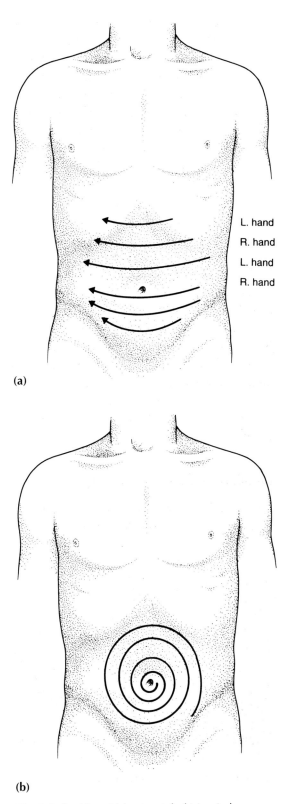

L. hand
R. hand
L. hand
R. hand

(a)

(b)

Fig. 8.6 Stroking: (a) horizontal; (b) in circles.

round the umbilicus. The circles should get larger so that initially you may be using only your fingers but will gradually use the whole hand (Fig. 8.6(b)).

Vibrations

Vibrations can be performed in three ways.

In walk standing facing across the model:

(1) With a flat hand over the area of the umbilicus, stationary vibration initially of small range and getting larger and deeper (i.e. of bigger amplitude).
(2) With flat hands following one another across the abdominal area in the same lines as stroking (Fig. 8.6(a)). This again can start gently and the amplitude can increase.

In walk standing at the level of the hips and facing the model:

(3) With a hand on each side behind the waist, vibrating stroking is performed quite strongly until the hands leave the abdomen. It is possible to continue the movement of the hands off the model to cross them and use them crossed. (Right hand on left waist and left hand on right waist.) The arms are uncrossed as this movement is completed. This is a deep manipulation and the sensation of lifting is imparted to the sides of the abdomen (Fig. 8.7(a) and (b)).

Stroking to the colon

The ascending colon

Cup the back of the right hand in the palm of the left hand and place the back of the left forearm near the elbow in the left iliac fossa.

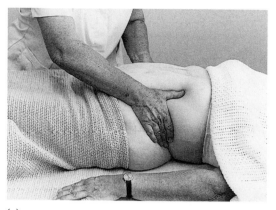

(a)

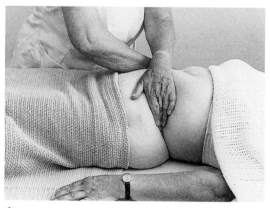

(b)

Fig. 8.7 Deep vibrating stroking: (a) start; (b) crossed hands.

Stroke with the backs of the left then right forearm upwards and outwards in the direction of the position of the ascending colon (Fig. 8.8(a), (b) and (c)).

The transverse colon

As you will not know where the transverse colon lies, its position being dependent on the contents and gravity, this is a continuation stroke to take the hands to the left side of the abdomen. As the hands leave the body after the ascending stroke and only the right forearm is in contact on the ascending stroke, the hands

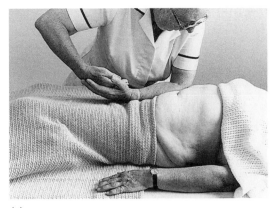

(a)

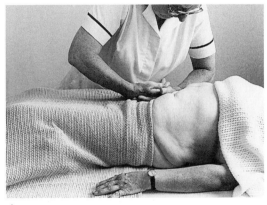

(b)

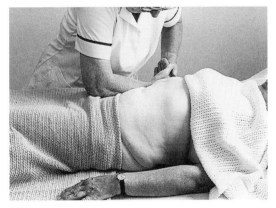

(c)

Fig. 8.8 Stroking for the colon: (a) start on the ascending colon; (b) continue upwards and outwards; (c) finish on the ascending colon.

are changed over so that the back of the left hand lies in the right palm. The right wrist leads the way across the abdomen to the left waist (Fig. 8.9(a)).

The descending colon

The hands are one on top of the other palm down with the right hand underneath. A deep stroke is performed from the left waist to the left iliac fossa. Greater depth is obtained if the thumb of the underneath (right) hand is

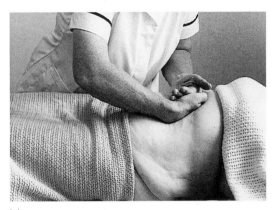

(a)

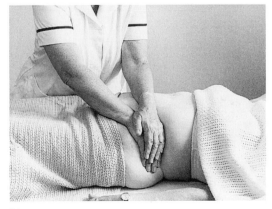

(b)

Fig. 8.9 Stroking for the colon: (a) the transverse colon – note the hands have changed over; (b) hands turned ready to work down the descending colon.

adducted and opposed so that it lies in the palm with the tip of the thumb over the proximal phalanx of the third and fourth digits (Fig. 8.9(a) and (b)).

Kneading to the colon

The ascending colon

Start in the right iliac fossa and work towards the waist using the right hand cupped so that the fingers are slightly elevated from the skin and the kneading is done with the palm. An upward and outward pressure is exerted while retaining the depth.

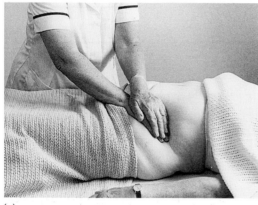

(a)

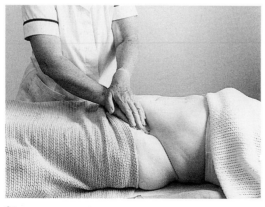

(b)

Fig. 8.10 Kneading the descending colon: (a) start; (b) note the depth.

The descending colon

Start at the left waist and work towards the left iliac fossa using the right hand. Narrow the hand by adducting and opposing the thumb into the palm. Exert downward and medial pressure while retaining the depth and finish with flat fingers as the palm has to be lifted to avoid the pubic area (Fig. 8.10(a) and (b)).

Rolling the colon

This manipulation can be performed if the content of the colon can be palpated as a sausage-like mass. The rolling is performed as in muscle rolling described in Chapter 2, but the area will be more circumscribed. Use the finger pads of both hands in line on one side of the mass and the thumbs in line on the other side of the mass. Roll gently forth and back and move on after a few manipulations. This manipulation can be used on both the descending and ascending colons (Fig. 8.11(a) and (b)).

Brisk lift stroking and shaking

Stand in walk standing facing the model. Place the hands one each side on the waist. Stroke deeply and very briskly inwards to midline so that the hands cross over to the other side. Put them crossed on the waist and stroke again deeply and briskly to uncross them. Repeat several times or intersperse with coarse vibrations done with the brisk strokes (Fig. 8.7(a) and (b)).

Skin wringing

This manipulation is performed by laying your hands on the abdomen and lifting the skin into your hands by pressure from both thumbs lying flat and tip to tip, and from the fingers lying with all four pads in line (Fig. 8.12). Once the

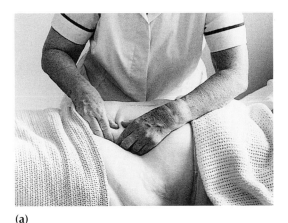

(a)

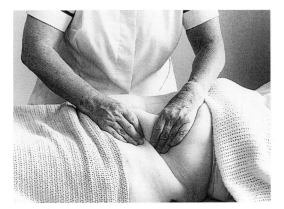

Fig. 8.12 Skin rolling the abdomen.

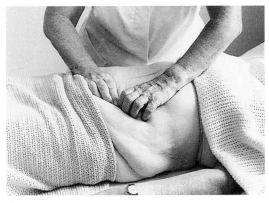

(b)

Fig. 8.11 Rolling the colon: (a) pull with the fingers; (b) push with the thumbs.

skin is lifted, a wringing manipulation is performed by bringing the fingers of one hand towards the thumb of the other hand.

Points to be observed

Abdominal massage can be performed at considerable depth once the patient is used to your hands. So always start more lightly and quickly work up to greater depth. Remember the contents of the abdomen are soft and can be moved by deeper manipulations, except where they are tied down to other organs as in the two fossae and at the flexures of the colon.

If the treatment is for constipation, the sequence of manipulations is:

(1) Palpation
(2) Whole abdomen stroking
(3) Whole abdomen kneading
(4) Stroking to the colon – starting with the descending colon
(5) Kneading to the colon – starting with the descending colon and possibly at the iliac fossa and working upwards to the splenic flexure. Then deal with the ascending colon, possibly starting at the hepatic flexure and working down to the iliac fossa.
(6) Rolling of the colon contents is done on the descending colon first, from below upwards, and then the ascending colon from above downwards
(7) Colon stroking is done again
(8) Finish with brisk lift stroking
(9) If the abdominal wall is flabby hacking may be performed in a pattern of vertical lines

Part II   SOME USES AND MODIFICATIONS FOR TREATMENT

Chapter 9
MASSAGE IN SPORT

Joan M. Watt

Massage has been used in sport from time immemorial. 'Athletes have resorted to massage since the days of the first Olympic Games, and the ancient athletes developed a special tool, the strygil, to scrape the masseur's oil from the skin' (Williams 1974).

Basic rules of sports massage

Before embarking on any description of sports massage, the basic rules of such a regime must be addressed:

(1) Diagnosis
(2) History
(3) Contra-indications
(4) Aims of treatment
(5) Position
(6) Materials
(7) Skin preparation
(8) Joint position
(9) Technique
(10) Check
(11) Clean up
(12) Warn patient

Diagnosis

Diagnosis will only apply if massage is being used to treat a sports injury. Many sports mas-

sages are classified as specific, i.e. not only to treat a particular problem but to help prepare prior to activity, between bouts of activity or after activity. Nonspecific sports massage is also used to help keep the body in tune.

History

It is always good practice to gain a full history, either relevant to a particular problem or previous experience of and reaction to massage.

Contra-indications

Contra-indications are as listed in Chapter 3. It is vitally important when dealing with sportspeople to remember the great risk of recent injury being present.

Aims of treatment

Is the massage to be stimulating or sedative? The aim of treatment will depend on when massage is to be administered, e.g. pre or post event.

Position

It cannot be guaranteed that there will always be a treatment couch available when using massage in sport. **Always** ensure that the therapist is going to be able to perform all necessary techniques with the greatest ease and that the recipient is at all times warm and comfortable.

Materials

Various oils may be used, most commonly vegetable based, ice and non-steroidal anti-inflammatory gel. Towels, ranging from small to very large, and inflatable pillows.

Skin preparation

Many sportspeople shave their legs before competition and small nicks are not unusual. Aseptic conditions should apply with absolute cleanliness essential.

Joint position

In the treatment rooms positioning as described in previous chapters should be adhered to. At track or pitch side be prepared to be innovative and use whatever is available and suitable to obtain the best joint position.

Technique

This will be addressed later in the chapter.

Check

Always ask the patient if the massage is deep enough, too deep, or as they want it.

Clean up

Participants cannot enter the competition arena covered in oil. A basketball player with oil on his thighs can get this on to his hands with disastrous results. Soap and water are available in the treatment room but not necessarily at pitch

side. In that situation wet-wipes or an astringent lotion should be available for use.

Warn participant

Even if the participant has frequent massages, always warn what to expect as a result of this session, e.g. pre-competition stimulating massage may induce a feeling of warmth but the rules of warm-up must still be observed.

Massage manipulations in sports massage

The massage manipulations used in sports massage are as described in Chapter 2, plus acupressure and ice massage.

Acupressure

Acupressure/acupuncture (acu is Chinese for needle) points are stimulated by finger or thumb pressure. There is a complete therapy using the 'tsubos' – specific sensitive points used in acupressure and also shiatsu (in Japanese shi = finger, atsu = pressure) where whole hands, elbows, feet and knees may be used to massage the body (Jarmey & Tindall 1991).

In sports massage acupressure tends to be to specific trigger points. These points are identified as tense, sometimes hard, and always producing pain in the muscle/connective tissue.

Once the point to be treated has been identified, the finger or thumb is used to apply pressure to that specific point. The technique is similar to that used in circular frictions but only one finger or the thumb tip is used. There are many different opinions as to the length of time the pressure should be held. A firm pressure accompanied with a slight circular motion applied for a maximum of one minute, relaxed and re-applied three or four times, gives good results. The object is to try to get muscle relaxation in as short a time as possible, thus making this technique very useful immediately prior to activity by removing particular spots of muscle/tissue tension. The use of both acupressure and shiatsu in sport is growing and there are many varying theories on the subjects, from basic applications to reduce muscle tensions right up to the complete science of the full holistic concept of Oriental medicine (Downer 1992).

Ice massage

The most convenient method of application of ice massage is to use a polystyrene cup which has been filled with water and then frozen. Cut a 1.25 cm ring from the top edge of the cup and then massage the injured area with the ice until an erythema is achieved. If dealing with tendinous or small areas an ice cube held in a tissue is best.

Sports massage

Sports massage can be divided into:

(1)   Specific sports massage
(2)   Non-specific sports massage

Specific sports massage

Specific sports massage is given for a particular reason and can be used in six different situations:

(1)   Massage in conditioning
(2)   Massage as treatment
(3)   Pre-competition massage
(4)   Inter-competition massage
(5)   Post competition massage
(6)   Post travel massage

These six specific sports massages may have to be carried out at pitch or track side and it may not always be possible to follow to the letter the manipulations, routines and methods suggested. The therapist must be prepared to be adaptable and use the manipulations and skills at his/her command in the most advantageous way to aid the participant in their chosen event.

Massage in conditioning

The conditioning time of year for any sportsperson will depend entirely on what their goals are for that particular year. The actual time of year will vary from sport to sport, dependent on the competitive season and major event(s). The object involves the SAID principle: Specific Adaptation Imposed Demands (Wallis & Logan 1964). This principle puts the body through safe and intense development, to achieve peak condition at the time of major competition. There may have to be more than one time of 'peaking' in each year, e.g. to qualify for Olympic selection in June and then to compete in the Olympic Games in September. Massage at the time of conditioning plays a very important part in the training regime.

Objects

(1)   **To promote recovery from a hard training session.** It is to be expected after a hard bout of exercise that the sportsperson will experience various aches, pains and a feeling of tired and heavy limbs. Massage can be invaluable in speeding up recovery at this time.

(2)   **To aid cool down.** The object of cool down is to return the body to its pre-exercise state as quickly and painlessly as possible. Massage at this time can be used to aid circulation, assist in the removal of waste products and enable the participant

to perform their cool down regimes more effectively.

(3) **To prevent delayed onset muscle soreness (DOMS).** It is widely appreciated that intense bouts of exercise will produce varying degrees of muscle soreness after the event. This soreness may not be noticed for up to 24 hours after cessation of the activity. Many learned sources will insist that there is no specific proof that massage will, in any way, prevent the occurrence of DOMS. On the other hand observation and anecdotal evidence lead those who are actively engaged in the field of sport massage to feel DOMS can be, and is, influenced positively by the application of the correct massage techniques.

(4) **Psychological effect.** The importance of the psychological effect of touch has never been fully quantified. At this hard time of training for the sportsperson a massage performed by a good knowledgeable practitioner can make a vast difference to their continued wellbeing and can enhance the benefits of the conditioning period.

Contact materials

Oils, mild warming rubs.

Routine and manipulations used

Light effleurage – accustoms the person to touch, also tests to see if there has been any micro trauma to soft tissue as a result of hard training.

Deep effleurage – to promote venous and lymphatic drainage.

Petrissage – to mobilise the soft tissues.

Deep effleurage – as above.

Acupressure – to address any specific tension or trigger spots identified.

Stroking – to provide relaxation and aid venous return.

Tapôtement/shaking/vibrations – to stimulate and give a feeling of wellbeing.

Effleurage – to aid venous and lymphatic return, and to assess the final state of the tissues.

Method

Start with the back, then the limbs, concentrating on the muscles most used in the training session. Often finish with a foot massage.

Duration

Whole body one to one and a half hours, half body half to three quarters of an hour. This massage can be given on a daily basis throughout the conditioning period, with the first massage being given the day before the first day of hard training.

Contra-indications

As described in Chapter 3, paying particular attention to identifying and avoiding any micro trauma that may have been occasioned by a particularly hard training session.

Massage as treatment

Massage as a treatment for sports injuries can be used after 48 hours if all bleeding and tissue swelling has ceased. In the case of haematoma, after four days or dependent on the patient's tolerance.

Objects

(1) **To stimulate circulation.** Forty eight hours after trauma it is important to clear away the debris of the incident and remove the

excess tissue fluid. Massage can play a useful part in reaching these goals.

(2) **To promote recovery from injury.** As stated above, to stimulate circulation and also to ensure the continued good state of surrounding tissues.

(3) **To break down adhesions.** The most important result after injury in sport must be that the individual has not been left with a tight shortened scar in any soft tissue. Adhesions and scar tissue are sources of trouble and can result in further trauma producing bigger and thicker areas of adherent tissue. Massage can play a very important part in the recovery.

(4) **To promote flexibility.** It is essential that all participants have returned at least to their previous level of flexibility after injury. Massage can provide a useful adjunct to the essential stretch routines performed by the patient.

(5) **To improve the range of movement.** Most types of injury, both soft tissue and bony, may well necessitate periods of strapping and/or immobilisation. A return to full range movement is necessary prior to return to full training and competition. Massage is used extensively to facilitate achieving a full range of movement.

Contact materials

Oil, cream, heat rub, ice, anti-inflammatory gel or cream.

Routine and manipulations used

Stroking – accustom the sportsperson to touch and discover any areas of sensitivity.

Effleurage – to promote venous and lymphatic return; depth will depend on injury.

Petrissage – to mobilise soft tissue and induce

slight stretch on those tissues; also to reduce muscle spasm.

Effleurage – as above.

Frictions – Counter-irritant effect as described in Chapter 2, to mobilise and break down scar tissue.

Tapôtement – excitation effect as described in Chapter 2, plus a feeling of wellbeing.

Effleurage – as above.

Shaking – applied both locally and to a total limb aids relaxation and relief of muscle tension and cramp. Acupressure – by stimulating trigger points it is possible to gain muscle relaxation or increase in muscle tone, dependent on depth and length of pressure applied.

Connective tissue massage – to mobilise the deep reticular layers of the dermis.

Rolling – as described in Chapter 2.

Effleurage – as above and to assess the final state of the tissues.

Method

Always massage proximal and then distal areas of the body before concentrating on the treatment area proper.

Duration

Dependent on area and sensitivity of the area to be treated – may be ten to thirty minutes. The treatment can be used daily depending on patient's level of discomfort and training/competition schedule.

Contra-indications

As described above, plus not within three days of training or competition if the methods are used to treat scar tissue or adhesions. Never if the patient cannot tolerate treatment.

Pre-competition massage

Massage prior to competition is to many sports-people part of the ritual carried out before their sporting endeavour. The time of this massage as part of the adjunct to performance must be carefully planned. If dealing with a team sport and all players require a massage, there must be adequate staff so that massages are not carried out many hours before the actual physical warm-up. In the case of individual performance, the report time and/or start time will decide the time of the pre-competition massage; for example: start time 10.30 AM, report time 10.10 AM, warm-up one hour, therefore the pre-competition massage must start at 8.40 AM at the latest.

Warm-up is the preparation of the body for physical activity. It is divided into three components:

(1)   Raising body temperature and increasing cardiovascular activity
(2)   Putting all joints through a full range of movement and all muscles into their greatest length of flexibility
(3)   Sport specific warm-up by practising the activities to be carried out.

Thus, a rugby player will end his/her warm-up with ball skills, passing and tackling; a hurdler will hurdle; and a discus thrower will practise the movements required to throw the discus.

This massage cannot be used instead of the participant's own physical warm-up but definitely can be used to enhance the preparation.

Objects

(1)   **To prepare muscles for exertion.** By increasing the circulation to specific areas and mobilising soft tissues. Massage prior to activity will make it easier to carry out the specific stretches needed for any performance.
(2)   **To aid warm-up effect.** As the term implies, warm-up is about warming the body prior to activity. The vasodilatation caused by massage will enhance this phase of physical preparation.
(3)   **Psychological effect.** The time spent on the massage couch is often used by participants to prepare mentally for the forthcoming action. This may be done in conversation with the therapist or may be inward and silent. There is a great advantage if the therapist knows the competitor well and knows whether or not they like to talk at this stage. It is also a good time to reinforce positive messages and allay fears about injury worries and the state of the opposition.

Contact materials

These must be carefully selected dependent on the activity about to take place and great care must be taken to clean the area well after the massage. Oils, creams, talcum are all appropriate, but do not use any heating agent. All rubefacients will cause vasodilatation of the skin and this will prove to be detrimental to the warm-up. The vasodilatation needs to be greatest below the dermis to aid warm-up.

Routine and manipulations used

Stroking – to accustom the person to touch.
Effleurage – to promote venous and lymphatic return, and discover any area which is particularly tight, tense, or giving pain.
Petrissage – to increase mobility of the soft tissues and stimulate circulation.

Tapôtement/shaking/vibration – all or one or two to promote feeling of wellbeing and give relief from muscle tension.

Effleurage – to finish massage and ascertain that the desired effects have been produced.

Trigger point acupressure – may be needed if there are specific areas of muscle spasm, tension or increased tone.

Method

As requested by the participant. Many sportspeople only want/need massage to a particular area, e.g. hamstrings or calf, while others request a full body massage.

Duration

Dependent on the area to be covered and length of time to achieve the desired effect of stimulation and to decrease any spasm or increased tone. Frequently 20–30 minutes but a maximum time of one hour. As a last minute attempt to decrease specific muscle tension, five minutes of acupressure can be used. It is best performed immediately prior to warm-up and it may well be followed by particular muscle stretch techniques such as contract/relax, stretch/relax as used in progressive neuromuscular facilitation techniques. **Do not use hot rubs.**

Contra-indications

As already stated and not if the competitor has not used massage prior to competition on previous occasions.

Inter-competition massage

When there is prolonged competition it will be necessary to provide inter-competition massage.

During a competition which has several rounds such as qualifying, quarter-final, semi-final and perhaps even finals on the same day, there are periods of rest in between. This is when massage can be very useful to the participant; also in multi-events at track and field, when the men do ten events over two days and the women seven. In this circumstance, if the athletes spent their normal time before and after each discipline doing warm-up and cool-down, they would be too tired to compete. Cool-down is the time immediately after training or competition when the participant will jog and perform specific exercises all aimed at returning the body to its resting state. Massage is extremely useful to complement a shortened warm-up and cool-down, but again cannot replace these essential activities. The only time massage can replace cool-down is if the participant is too exhausted to perform an active cool-down or if injury precludes activity. **Massage can never replace active warm-up.**

Objects

(1) **To promote recovery.** After a bout of exercise there will be waste products in the tissues. Massage, by stimulating venous and lymphatic return, aids the process of elimination of such products.

(2) **To refresh the competitor.** In a prolonged competition it is not unusual to experience muscle fatigue and general tiredness. Stimulating massage can be advantageous to combat both feelings.

(3) **To work out niggles.** After hard exercise there may well be a feeling of tightness in certain muscle groups, which will not respond to the competitor's normal series of stretching exercises. Massage can be used to help physically and also to reassure

the participant that there is no major problem developing.

(4) **To prevent muscle cramps and spasms.** It is not unusual, especially if the competition is taking place in a situation where dehydration can occur, to be presented with cramps. While the competitor rehydrates with the correct fluids, massage can be used to help increase the circulation to the affected part.

Contact materials

Be careful to select the correct medium. If the area is sweaty or has sand or chalk on it, it must first be cleansed. The pores will be open and you do not want to clog these with any medium which will impede heat loss. A very light oil or soapy water is best. Never use any hot rubs at this stage. It may be necessary to use ice massage if there is an area where there could be actual tissue damage.

Routine and manipulations used

Stroking – to accustom the person to touch and to assess the temperature and state of the area to be massaged.

Effleurage – to promote venous and lymphatic return and discover any particularly tense spot(s).

Petrissage – to help remove the waste products and mobilise the soft tissues. The rolling manipulations described in Chapter 2 are particularly useful here.

Acupressure – to any area which is excessively tense or tending to cramp.

Vibrations and shaking – whole limb shaking and vibration are very good towards the end of this massage to ensure the limb is ready for the next bout of exerise and unlikely to go into cramp.

Effleurage – to complete the session and prepare the competitor for their warm-up.

Method

As needed by the competitor. Early on in the day the request may be to address one specific area that is bothering the competitor. But as the competition continues and usually before and/or after the last event of the day, it may be necessary to cover the full body.

Duration

As time allows; may be for only several minutes or up to an hour. It is best to perform inter-competition massage immediately after cool-down and/or prior to the next warm-up.

Contra-indications

As previously stated, and any area of recent trauma must be avoided.

Post competition massage

At the cessation of activity the competitor will do cool-down. Massage can be used to enhance the effects of this procedure. On certain occasions it may be necessary to replace active cool-down with massage and passive movements, e.g. after a marathon, long distance event, or when the competitor has sustained an injury which precludes active cool-down.

Objects

(1) **To carry away waste products** – as used in inter-competition massage.

(2) **To allow body functions to return to normal.** At the end of any period of physical activity the cardiovascular system may be working excessively hard, or as a result of the cessation of activity the blood pressure can suddenly drop. Massage, especially centripetal effleurage, is very useful in restoring normality.

(3) **To prevent post-exercise pain** – as previously described in massage in conditioning.

(4) **To work out niggles.** Frequently after activity the participant may complain of certain specific areas of pain or tension. If any tissue damage is suspected, ice massage can be applied. If the cause is purely exercise induced, then massage is beneficial to remove the tightness.

(5) **Psychological effect.** As previously described this can be very important either if the competitor is on a 'high' after competing successfully or, conversely, 'down' after a poor performance.

Contact materials

Ice, soapy water, light oil but not any hot rubs or talcum.

Routine and manipulations used

All manipulations to be used slowly and rhythmically. Stroking – to assess the area and accustom the sportsperson to touch.

Effleurage – at first light and centripetal, then deeper if there is no tension or pain. It can be performed in all directions, to increase circulation and remove waste products.

Petrissage – starting fairly light and deepening to a level the participant can tolerate.

Effleurage – interspersed between all other strokes and for at least five minutes at the end of the massage to enhance tissue drainage.

Method

As requested by the competitor, may be only to one specific area or may be to whole body area and in some instances may be used in place of active cool-down.

Duration

Dependent on the area to be covered it may last 15–30 minutes or may take a full hour. This massage is best performed after the active cool-down and preceded by a tepid shower. When taking the place of an active cool-down it is essential to ensure that the participant is adequately rehydrating as well as receiving massage.

Contra-indications

Again as previously described, and being very circumspect around painful areas which might well be caused by micro trauma, in which case only ice massage should be applied.

Post travel massage

It is very common for all types of sportspeople to have to travel varying distances to participate in competition all over the world. Wherever possible sufficient time should be allowed to permit adequate acclimatisation both to time change and climatic conditions. In reality the competitors may not be able to allow this time to adjust. The length of time spent on travel and the frequency of this travel can adversely affect performance.

Travel problems highlighted in sport are:

- General feeling of stiffness
- Feeling of lassitude
- Aches, especially in the lower back, neck and shoulders
- Swelling of lower legs and feet

Solutions are:

- Light exercise
- Shower
- Jacuzzi
- Massage

Objects

(1) **To increase the venous and lymphatic flow,** thus removing swelling and stiffness.
(2) **Gently and deeply to stretch the soft tissues,** to remove aches and increase flexibility.
(3) **To remove any residual stiffness** without tiring the competitor with exercise.
(4) **To restore the normal balance of the body.**
(5) **To create a feeling of wellbeing.**

Contact materials

Oil or creams. Do not use talcum or hot rubs as there may well be some dehydration present.

Routine and manipulations used

Stroking – to assess the condition of the skin and accustom to touch.

Effleurage – first centripetal to aid tissue drainage and increase venous and lymphatic return. Then multi-directional to promote tissue stretching.

Petrissage – especially kneading, wringing, picking up and rolling techniques to assist drainage and stretch the soft tissues.

Effleurage – should be interspersed regularly with all other strokes.

Tapôtement, vibration and shaking – to aid venous and lymphatic return and to promote a feeling of wellbeing.

Method

Start with the back and neck, then the legs and if necessary the arms as well. Finish with assisted stretches to the major muscle groups used in the participant's activity.

Duration

Dependent on the areas to be covered. A minimum of 30 minutes but may last over an hour. Best results are gained if the participant has already carried out some gentle activity, such as a jog and gentle stretches, and then had a tepid shower prior to massage.

Contra-indications

As previously described, paying particular attention to the effects of dehydration.

Non-specific sports massage

There are times in the competitor's year when there is no competition or conditioning taking place. At those times the athlete will still be maintaining his/her body in a state of pre-paredness for the activities of the future. Massage can play a very important and helpful part at those times and is referred to as non-specific massage. This term also applies to massage given when the competitor has arrived at the competition site ahead of the event by at least two days, or finished competition and is still present at the competition site, waiting for the rest of the team to complete com-petition and return home. Basically we are referring to a massage which is given for no specific treatment purpose, and is not before, between or after competition or travel. Non-specific sports massage can be divided into two applications:

(1) General body massage
(2) Specific areas of massage

General body massage

Sportspeople spend a large part of their lives conditioning and preparing their bodies for the rigours of their particular sport. Many of them firmly believe that regular full body massage will aid them in their pursuit of excellence.

Objects

(1) **To enhance a general feeling of wellbeing**
(2) **To promote relaxation** if this is desired by the participant
(3) **To stimulate** if requested by the participant
(4) **To monitor** the condition of the musculature and soft tissues
(5) **To highlight** and deal with any area which could develop into a problem

Contact materials

Oils. If knowledgeable, aromatherapy can be used (see Chapter 10), creams, mild warming rub, talcum powder.

Routine and manipulations used

For objects 1 and 2:
    Stroking – to accustom to touch.
    Effleurage – long slow manipulations used continuously.
    Kneading – deep enough not to tickle, slow and rhythmical.
    Effleurage – slow to end the session.
For objects 1 and 3:
    As described in precompetition massage.
For object 4:
    Deep effleurage.
For object 5:
    Trigger pointing and friction may be added and in this case the non-specific massage will change to a treatment massage if specific problem areas are highlighted.

Method

For objects 1 and 2, as described in Chapter 2, starting with back and neck, then each limb in turn, foot massage as opposed to facial massage and, if deemed necessary, finish by returning to the back.

For objects 1 and 3, as described in precompetition massage.

For object 4, extra effleurage at the start and finish of the session.

For object 5, as described in treatment massage.

Duration

For objects 1 and 2, as long as is needed to gain desired relaxation, usually an hour to an hour and a half. It is important that the competitor can lie and relax for at least half an hour after completion of the massage.

For objects 1 and 3, as described in precompetition massage.

For object 4, a few extra moments at the end of each session.

For object 5, as your findings necessitate.

Contra-indications

As previously described.

Specific areas of massage

Dependent on the muscle groups most used in their particular event, the competitor may request an area of body to receive massage, rather than a full body, e.g. throwers – back and/or shoulders; sprinters – hamstrings, quadriceps and calf muscles; distance events and soccer players – calf massage.

Objects, contact materials and manipulations

As described in general body massage.

Method

Concentrate on the area highlighted by the participant but do not forget to clear the surrounding area.

Duration

As long as is needed to gain the desired effects.

Contra-indications

As previously described.

Summary

- **Never give a first massage to a participant within 48 hours of competition**
- Arrange for the first massage to take place when there is plenty of time for any adverse effects to be worked off
- Adverse effects may be
  - producing too much relaxation
  - stirring up old problems such as scar tissue

Sports massage may be sport specific and any therapist involved must know and understand the principles of that sport. Most importantly, the rules and call-up times of the sport must be understood. As already stated, there will not always be time to perform the beginning, middle and end of a massage as you might wish. The most important issue in a situation where time is of the essence is to be absolutely clear about the main object of this massage. It may be to eliminate a particular point of tension or increase range of movement. Having identified the object, choose which of the techniques can best deliver the desired effect and use them. If the sport is an outdoor activity it may not even be possible to remove clothing, e.g. skiing, orienteering, distance running - participants frequently wear tights or jogging bottoms to protect their legs. In instances like these whole limb shaking, vibration or trigger pointing through the clothing will be the best massage techniques to use.

References

Downer, J. (1992) *Headway Lifeguides*. Hodder & Stoughton, London.

Jarmey, C. & Tindall, J. (1991) *Acupressure for Common Ailments*. Gaia Books, London.

Wallis, E.L. & Logan, G.A. (1964) *Figure Improvement and Body Conditioning Through Exercise*. Prentice Hall, New York.

Williams, J. (1974) *Massage and Sport*. Bayer, Switzerland.

Chapter 10
MASSAGE AND ITS USES IN AROMATHERAPY

Elizabeth Jones

Introduction to aromatherapy

Aromatherapy may be defined as a therapeutic procedure which utilises the fragrant substances extracted from aromatic plants. The fragrant substances generally used by aromatherapists are the essential oils of these plants.

Historical uses of essential oils

Since time immemorial aromatic plants and their extracts have been used for religious, medicinal and cosmetic purposes.

Egyptians: 3000–1500 BC

The ancient Egyptians not only used them for religious rites (embalming of bodies, using in particular cedarwood oil), but also for their therapeutic effects (fragrant unguents on sun-baked skin to soothe and maintain elasticity). A famous perfume, *Kyphi*, was made of a mixture of fragrant herbs and resins. Plutarch said that the aromatic substances included in the perfume Kyphi 'lulled one to sleep, allayed anxieties and brightened dreams' (Genders 1972).

Greeks: 500–40 BC

The Greeks also used aromatics for medicinal as well as for body-enhancing purposes. A famous Greek perfume *Megaleion*, named after its Greek creator Megallus, was used not only for its scent but also for healing wounds and reducing inflammation.

Europeans: 12th Century

Many monasteries had their own aromatic herb gardens and used the plants and extracts to heal the sick who came to their doors. Abbess Hildegard of Bingen is known to have utilised both the plant and the essential oil of lavender.

Europeans: 16th Century

To ward off the plague, according to a book written in French, *Les Secrets de Maitre Alexis de Piedmont*, the house should be fumigated with all manner of fragrant substances including rosemary, cloves, nutmeg, sage, aloes and juniper wood (Genders 1972).

Europeans: 17th Century

By the beginning of the 17th Century approximately 60 oils were being used for their perfume and medicinal effects (Valnet 1980).

Europeans: 19th Century

'The first research into the antiseptic powers of essential oils was undertaken by Chamberland in 1887 in his work on the anthrax bacillus. He noted the active properties of origanum, Chinese cinnamon, Singhalese cinnamon, angelica and Algerian geranium' (Valnet 1980).

Europeans: 20th Century

Cavel's research on microbic cultures in sewage has shown many essences to have infertilising properties at considerable dilutions (Valnet 1980). Cavel in fact researched 35 oils, finding thyme, origanum and sweet orange the most effective (Cavel 1918).

Gattefose, a French chemist, was the person who first coined the term aromatherapy, having during and after World War I made an extensive study of the use of essence, and published a book called *Aromatherapy* in 1937.

During World War 2, Dr Jean Valnet, another Frenchman, inspired by Gattefosse's work, started to use essential oils in his clinical practice. His medication included both internal and external methods of use.

By the 1960s a small band of enthusiasts (the foremost being Madame Maury, a French bio-chemist) began to incorporate essential oils into massage treatments. This use of essential oils has grown steadily and aromatherapy massage, when given by properly qualified practitioners, is now widely used in hospitals, hospices and clinics.

Essential oils

An essential oil may be defined as an odorous, volatile substance, present within all aromatic plant matter. In many cases the amount is so minute that it is not practicable, or is too expensive, to isolate it. Essential oils are not confined to flowers. They may be found in leaves, grasses, seeds, roots, rhizomes and fruits as well as woods and resins.

When essential oils are produced in more than one part of a plant, the individual oils will differ in composition and fragrance, e.g. the bitter orange tree gives a bitter orange oil from the rind of the orange, the petitgrain oil from the leaves and the green twigs and the neroli oil from its freshly picked flowers.

Basic chemistry

'A typical essential oil is a complex mixture of chemical compounds, each of which possesses its own individual properties' (Williams 1989).

'All of the constituents of an essential oil are organic; that is, their molecular structures are based upon arrangements of carbon atoms blended into one another and to atoms of hydrogen. Oxygen atoms are present in many of the constituents of essential oils and sometimes atoms of nitrogen and/or sulphur' (Williams 1989).

The constituents which have molecules containing carbon and hydrogen only are called hydrocarbons.

Terpenes

The hydrocarbons found in essential oils are called terpenes, which are 'unsaturated' hydrocarbons as their molecules do not have the maximum number of hydrogen atoms it would be possible for them to contain. As a result they easily combine with atoms of oxygen in the air. The terpenes are divided into three types:

(1) Mono-terpenes – which have 10 carbon atoms
(2) Sesqui-terpenes – which have 15 carbon atoms
(3) Di-terpenes – which have 20 carbon atoms

Oxygenated compounds

The constituents of essential oils which have oxygen as well as hydrogen and carbon in their molecular structure are called oxygenated compounds. They have varied characteristics and among the different types are alcohols, phenols, aldehydes, esters, lactones and ketones.

The number of constituents in an essential oil varies but there may be 100 or more when analysed. The contribution of any one constituent to the unique scent of an essential oil depends on:

(1) The proportion of the constituent
(2) The volatility of the constituent
(3) The quality of the constituent
(4) The strength of odour of the constituent

The varying evaporation rates of the individual constituents will affect the fragrance of the essential oil over the passage of time. 'It is the odours of the oxygenated constituents and to a secondary degree the odours of their sesquiterpenes which determine the odours of almost all the essential oils' (Williams 1989).

Effects on mind and body

A perfume uses natural and synthetic materials to combine odour and volatility to give the wearer maximum psychological pleasure from the fragrance which he/she has chosen. This pleasure results from the stimulation of the olfactory nerve endings in the nose. An aromatherapist combines psychological with physiological effects to gain maximum therapeutic value from the essential oils.

Aromatherapists remain firmly committed to using only natural essential oils from aromatic plants. According to one writer 'it has been demonstrated that the anti-inflammatory and other medicinal properties of some natural oils, some of which have been used since Biblical times, are gentler and less toxic than the pure active drugs isolated from the oil' (van Toller & Dodd 1988). These essential oils offer a state of wellbeing not only for the mind but also for the body.

Extraction methods

Distillation

Distillation is the method usually employed for extracting the essential oil from a plant.

Expression

The expression technique is reserved for citrus oils because they are unable to withstand the rigours of distillation.

Solvent extraction

Aromatic extracts such as concretes and absolutes and resinoids contain considerable amounts of non-volatile matter and cannot therefore be truly termed essential oils. They are removed by chemical solvents from the plant matter which stores them. They are sometimes used by aromatherapists. Figure 10.1 shows aromatic derivatives from plants.

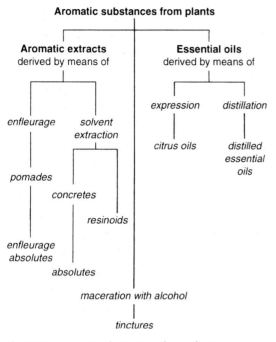

Fig. 10.1 Aromatic derivatives from plants.

Enfleurage

This method used to be used to extract absolutes for perfumery. Glass plates were covered with a film of cold fat on which fragrant flower petals were laid, their essential oils being absorbed by the fat.

Maceration

Some essential oils are too difficult or too costly to distil and are therefore extracted by a method called maceration. Plants such as calendula, lime blossom and melissa are cut up and placed in a vat of vegetable oil, e.g. almond or sunflower, and agitated for some days. The molecules of the essential oils are absorbed by the vegetable oil, the liquid filtered and then bottled.

Purity of essential oils

Essential oils used by aromatherapists for therapeutic massage should be of the highest quality, and of natural not synthetic origin. The quality of the oil will depend on the good reputation of a high grade supplier. The supplier will have had the oils tested in a variety of ways before marketing them. Tests may include:

(1) The specific gravity (SG) test
(2) The refractive index test
(3) Capillary gas/liquid chromatography test
(4) Triangle test

In this way adulteration, ageing and change of proportion of constituent compounds of the oil may be checked, and only the finest oils sold.

Storage

Essential oils can deteriorate rapidly. It is very important therefore that they are stored under the following conditions:

(1) They should be in containers which will not interact with the oil. Glass is usual for small amounts. Internally lacquered steel drums are used for amounts over 10 kg. Plastic containers are no good as the plastic and oil interact.
(2) The containers should be sealed very well.
(3) The containers should be protected from light, particularly from strong sunlight because it has a chemical catalytic effect (photocatalytic) which precipitates chemical changes in the oil. Artificial light is not so damaging.
(4) They should be kept in cool conditions. Almost all oils can be kept in a refrigerator at 5°C. Vetivert, sandalwood, cedarwood and patchouli should be kept at a

room temperature of 15°C. Rose oil, rose absolute and some other oils will solidify but this is no problem as they will re-melt at room temperature. Under no circumstances should they be heated.

(5) For the therapist running a clinic it is sensible to order only small quantities, to avoid deterioration.

Most commonly used essential oils

It is important that an aromatherapist has a working knowledge of the traditional uses of at least 40 oils (see Table 10.1). The more usual essential oils are:

basil	*Ocimum basilicum*
benzoin	*Styrax benzoin*
bergamot	*Citrus bergamia*
cajeput	*Melaleuca cajeputi*
cedarwood	*Cedrus virginia*
	Cedrus atlantica
chamomile	
Moroccan	*Ormenis multicaulis*
Roman	*Chamaemelum nobile*
clary sage	*Salvia sclarea*
cypress	*Cupressus sempervirens*
eucalyptus	*Eucalyptus globulus*
fennel	*Foeniculum vulgaris*
frankincense	*Boswellia carteri*
geranium	*Pelargonium graveolens*
ginger	*Zingiber officianalis*
hyssop	*Hyssopus officianalis*
jasmine	*Jasminum officianale*
juniper	*Juniper communis*
lavender	*Lavender angustifolia*
lemon	*Citrus limon*
lemon balm	*Melissa officianalis*
lemongrass	*Cymbopogon citratus*
mandarin	*Citrus reticulata*
marjoram (sweet)	*Origanum marjorana*
myrrh	*Commiphora myrrha*

myrtle	*Myrtus communis*
neroli	*Citrus aurantium*
niaouli	*Melaleuca viridiflora*
peppermint	*Mentha piperita*
orange, sweet	*Citrus aurentium*
patchouli	*Pogostemon cablin*
pepper (black)	*Piper nigrum*
pine	*Pinus sylvestris*
rose	*Rosa centrifolia*
	Rosa damascena
rosemary	*Rosmarinus officianalis*
sage	*Salvia lavendulaefolia*
sandalwood	*Santalum album*
teatree	*Melaleuca alternifolia*
thyme	*Thymus vulgaris*
ylang ylang	*Cananga odorata, var. genuina*

Therapeutic use of essential oils

Ingestion

Essential oils may be administered orally, or via the anus or vagina. However this is a form of treatment which should only be undertaken by those qualified in a field such as phytotherapy because this method carries the greatest risks of adverse effects. Though some doctors in France specialise in treatment by ingestion, it is rarely used in this way in the UK or the US. Aromatherapists therefore generally administer essential oils therapeutically via olfaction, inhalation and skin absorption. (See Fig. 10.2 later for methods of use and passage of essentials into the body.)

Olfaction

Olfaction occurs when the sense of smell is interpreted by the olfactory apparatus. This starts in the nose where the olfactory receptors are situated, and travels via impulses along the

Table 10.1

Term	Property	Essential oil
Analgesic	gives pain relief	basil, benzoin, bergamot, black pepper, cajeput, camphor, chamomile, clary sage, coriander, cypress, eucalyptus, geranium, ginger, juniper, lavender, lemon, lemongrass, marjoram, melissa, orange, peppermint, pine, rosemary, sage, thyme
Anticontusive	prevents bruises	geranium, ginger, hyssop
Antidepressant	counters low spirits	bergamot, camphor, chamomile, clary sage, coriander, geranium, jasmine, lavender, melissa, neroli, orange, patchouli, pine, rose, sage, sandalwood, thyme, ylang ylang
Antifungal		myrrh, teatree
Antiseptic	inhibits growth of bacteria	almost all oils
Antispasmodic	relieves smooth muscle spasm	basil, bergamot, cajeput, camphor, chamomile, coriander, cypress, eucalyptus, fennel, frankincense, geranium, hyssop, jasmine, juniper, lavender, mandarin, marjoram, melissa, black pepper, peppermint, rose, rosemary, sage, sandalwood, thyme
Antiphlogistic	reduces inflammation and vasoconstricts	benzoin, chamomile, clary sage, cypress, geranium, jasmine, lavender, myrrh, neroli, niaouli, peppermint, rose, sandalwood.
Antiviral		niaouli, teatree
Aphrodisiac	increases sexual desire	clary sage, jasmine, neroli, patchouli, black pepper, rose, sandalwood, ylang ylang
Astringent	tightens tissues	bergamot, camphor, cedarwood, frankincense, geranium, juniper, lemon, patchouli, rose, rosemary, sage, sandalwood
Carminative	eases bowel pain and expels wind	basil, bergamot, black pepper, camphor, chamomile, coriander, fennel, ginger, hyssop, juniper, lavender, mandarin, melissa, myrrh, neroli, peppermint, rosemary, sage, sandalwood, thyme
Cordial	acts as a tonic for the heart	benzoin, camphor, lavender, lemon, mandarin, rosemary
Cytophylactic	stimulates cell regeneration	almost all oils
Depurative	purifies the blood of toxins and waste	eucalyptus, hyssop, jasmine, juniper, rose
Digestive	aids digestion	basil, bergamot, cajeput, camphor, chamomile, geranium, ginger, hyssop, lemongrass, marjoram, myrrh, orange, thyme
Diuretic	removes fluid from the body through the kidneys	camphor, cedarwood, chamomile, cypress, eucalyptus, fennel, frankincense, geranium, juniper, lavender, lemon, marjoram, orange, patchouli, black pepper, pine, rosemary, sage, sandalwood, thyme

Table 10.1 *Continued*

Term	Property	Essential oil
Emmenagogue	menstrual problems	basil, cajeput, chamomile, clary sage, cypress, fennel, ginger, hyssop, jasmine, juniper, lavender, marjoram, melissa, myrrh, peppermint, rose, rosemary, sage, sandalwood, thyme, ylang ylang
Euphoric	uplifts into an excited state	clary sage, ylang ylang
Expectorant	expels mucus from the chest	basil, benzoin, cedarwood, cypress, eucalyptus, frankincense, hyssop, lemon, myrrh, niaouli, peppermint, sandalwood, thyme
Febrifuge	reduces fever	camphor, chamomile, cypress, eucalyptus, hyssop, lemongrass, melissa, orange, black pepper, peppermint
Haemostatic	arrests bleeding	geranium, rose
Hyperpnoea	reduces abnormally fast breathing	ylang ylang
Hepatic	helps with liver problems	chamomile, mandarin, peppermint, rose, rosemary
Hypotensor	reduces blood pressure	clary sage, hyssop, lavender, lemon, marjoram, melissa, ylang ylang
Hypertensor	raises blood pressure	mandarin, rosemary, sage, thyme
Laxative	helps to evacuate bowels	camphor, fennel, ginger, hyssop, mandarin, orange, black pepper, rose
Nervine	useful for nervous disorders in general	basil, cedarwood, chamomile, coriander, cypress, hyssop, juniper, lavender, lemon, lemongrass, mandarin, melissa, orange, peppermint, rosemary, thyme
Rubefacient	stimulates circulation	benzoin, camphor, coriander, eucalyptus, juniper, lemon, black pepper, peppermint, pine, rosemary, sage, thyme
Sedative	soothes the nervous system	benzoin, bergamot, camphor, cedarwood, chamomile, clary sage, cypress, frankincense, geranium, hyssop, jasmine, juniper, lavender, marjoram, melissa, neroli, patchouli, peppermint, rose, sandalwood, ylang ylang
Stimulant	has a tonic action on mind and body	coriander, eucalyptus, hyssop, jasmine, lemon, niaouli, orange, black pepper, pine, rosemary, sage
Tonic	mild astringent	lemon, mandarin, sage
Vulnerary	heals sores and wouds	benzoin, cajeput, camphor, chamomile, eucalyptus, frankincense, geranium, hyssop, jasmine, juniper, lavender, lemon, orange, patchouli, rosemary, sandalwood, thyme

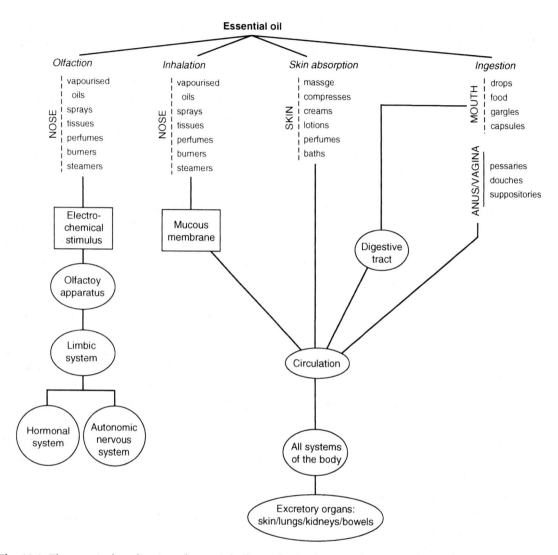

Fig. 10.2 The practical application of essential oils: methods of use, and passage of essential oils in the body.

olfactory nerve (CI) to the olfactory bulbs on the underside of the brain. There are two groups of receptor cells of about 25 million each, which lie in a small area at the top of the nose. Protruding from the cells are olfactory hairs which are so small as to be visible only when very highly magnified by an electron microscope; they lie immersed in the thin watery secretion of the mucus which covers the surfaces of the nasal cavities (Williams 1989).

Odour molecules from the essential oils are volatile, and fat and water soluble. 'As a result when we breathe in these molecules they easily penetrate the mucus layer and come into contact with the olfactory cilia. The incoming molecules fit into the receptor sites and initiate an electrochemical reaction in a "lock and key" action' (Vickers 1996a).

The olfactory apparatus is closely associated with the limbic system (hippocampus and amygdala), once known as the rhinen-cephalen or 'nose-brain'. The limbic system is that part of the brain which is concerned with feelings, emotions, moods and motivation. It influences eating, aggressive action and sexual activity and controls certain hormones and the autonomic nervous system. There is quite a lot of observational evidence which shows that odours influence mind and body, e.g. menstrual synchrony in female humans is thought to be due to odour (Schwartz & Natyncuk 1990), and the insect world communicates by the volatile chemical pheromones.

The fragrance of essential oils transmitted via the olfactory system to specialised areas of the brain undoubtedly creates psychological effects which in turn may achieve physical effects of a therapeutic nature.

Inhalation

Inhalation occurs when we breathe air into the lungs. When the vapour from an essential oil containing aromatic molecules passes into the respiratory system it can have an effect throughout the system. Many traditional remedies advocate the use of essential oils in boiling water and in vaporising chest rubs to improve respiratory function. Clinical tests have been carried out which support the use of such inhalations (Berger *et al.* 1978; Saller *et al.* 1990).

The aromatic molecules also pass through the walls of the alveoli in the lungs and enter the bloodstream. Again, clinical research has shown this to happen. Among those who have done such tests are Kovar *et al.* (1987), Buchbauer *et al.* (1993) and Falk-Filipsson (1993).

Skin absorption

Until relatively recently it was thought that the skin was virtually impermeable, but it is now known that the skin and mucous membranes are able to absorb lipophilic substances (Brun 1952).

Traditionally, the action of oils when they are absorbed through the skin is considered to be similar to when they are absorbed into the capillary network around the alveoli of the lungs. They enter the bloodstream and are transported round the body until naturally eliminated.

Whether absorbed by the lungs or skin it is possible they influence the body processes. Some may stimulate the release of endorphins – the body's own chemicals which can have an analgesic or anti-depressant effect – some appear to have a diuretic effect, while others may be able to help with hormonal balances of the body or support the immune system.

Just as oils work on the respiratory tissue itself during inhalation, so essences can have an effect on the skin itself during skin absorption. Essential oils therefore not only provide pleasing fragrances, which have an effect on the mind, but can have beneficial effects on the body also.

Terms and properties of some essential oils

The terminology applied to the uses of essential oils has been borrowed from herbal medicine. A list of such terms together with the properties of some essential oils is given in Table 10.1.

Practical application of essential oils

Figure 10.2 illustrates the different methods by which essential oils may be utilised for therapeutic purposes, and their passage into the body.

The holistic approach

There are various ways of viewing the cause and treatment of disease. It is held that conventional medicine locates all disease in the physical body; even emotional distress is viewed as a biochemical disorder that requires biochemical intervention. Holistic medicine seeks the roots and treatment of disease, not just in the individual's body but also in the mind, family, environment and community. In cancer, for instance, it has been claimed that an individual's temperament (Eysenck 1988) and social family links (Reynolds *et al.* 1994) affect the onset of disease (Vickers 1996b).

The practical application of essential oils for therapeutic purposes uses the holistic approach both during consultation and in treatment. Aromatherapy is considered to be one of the complementary therapies, but its usefulness in the treatment of many conditions is now widely appreciated by those working in orthodox medicine. Consequently an ever increasing number of doctors, nurses, physiotherapists and other para-medical workers are including aromatherapy as part of the 'care package' they offer in hospitals, hospices and clinics.

Aromatherapy massage

The combination of the therapeutic effects of essential oils with the therapeutic effects of the 'laying on' of hands, namely massage, provides a 'natural' treatment of considerable value. Not only are the oils utilised by skin absorption, but also by olfaction and inhalation, when applied by massage.

Aromatherapy massage probably creates the most diffuse therapeutic effect, if compared with other methods of use of essential oils. It is also a very safe treatment when practised by a competent and well trained, qualified aromatherapist.

The massage techniques described in this book which would be the most appropriate are effleurage (stroking) and petrissage (kneading). Many aromatherapists, myself included, use further techniques such as lymphatic drainage and neuro-muscular and acupressure manipulations of the soft tissue.

Lymphatic drainage

These manipulations involve short or long, light or deep stroking movements which help move on excess fluids, waste matter and toxins, through the lymphatic system towards the heart and into the general circulation, and thence to the excretory organs of the body.

Neuro-muscular massage

These manipulations involve a knowledge of the relationship between the cutaneous sensory zones of the body, the autonomic nervous system and the internal organs. Movements include deep palmar kneadings and deep finger kneadings in the zones.

Acupressure massage

These manipulations include a knowledge of the philosophies of acupuncture and shiatsu. The movements include working with thumbs on meridians (energy lines) and tsubo points (areas where energy blockages may be released).

Effects and uses of aromatherapy massage

My own experience, and that of many aromatherapists, has shown that aromatherapy massage is the most popular form of treatment with essential oils. There are a number of consistent themes in the experience of, and response to, massage and aromatherapy in different client groups. Patients report that they feel better after aromatherapy massage and this is an important consequence in many conditions.

Cancer care

Aromatherapy reportedly relieves the symptoms of fatigue and the stress to which such patients are subject. It may also have a short-term effect on the musculo-skeletal pain and is often used in hospices. It is especially useful when one-to-one care is given.

Infections

Some essential oils are specifically anti-microbial and some people claim there can be an effect on the immune system. There is especial interest in this context in its use for the treatment of those with AIDS.

Physically and mentally disabled children

Aromatherapy is used for its relaxing effect and for its anti-microbial effects as well as for relief of musculo-skeletal pain.

Stress and anxiety

Used both as a skin application by massage and self-administered in the bath or by inhalation, aromatic oils are said to help patients gain a feeling of relaxation.

Insomnia

Sleep may be induced by the use of an aromatherapy massage.

Long stay in bed or in a wheelchair

Aromatherapy massage may help to prevent pressure sores by enhancing the circulation to those body parts subject to pressure (Vickers 1996b).

Pregnancy/childbirth/babycare

Aromatherapy massage can help pain and insomnia and give a sense of deep relaxation. It is therefore of considerable benefit to those who are pregnant, in labour, or have post-natal depression.

Massage for babies is common in certain countries and the use of essential oils with massage for babies is becoming widespread in the western countries. It helps the 'bonding' process between parent and child, and may increase the child's resistance to infection, improve weight gain and help general mental and physical development.

Older people

Aromatherapy massage is being used more widely in the care of older people. This is a time of life when people may feel especially alone, depressed and fearful. Aromatherapy massage to hands, feet, neck and shoulders can help to break the sense of isolation and inspire calm and peace. Other problems which may be helped are:

(1) Pain in the musculo-skeletal system
(2) Constipation
(3) Dyspepsia
(4) Insomnia
(5) Pressure sores

Consultation procedures

As aromatherapy is a holistic therapy, the consultation procedure should take a full 25–30 minutes. Different aromatherapists will approach a consultation in a variety of ways, but all well qualified professionals will seek to discover a complete picture of the events leading to the patient's condition. This will include such areas as their medical, social and family background.

The patient consultation is a vital prelude to a session of treatments. It leads to correct assessment both physical and psychological, and therefore to correct treatment. My approach is to use three major techniques:

(1) Verbal
(2) Visual
(3) Tactile

The first very important point of communication is when the patient makes a booking, by telephone or by coming to the clinic. It is very important that they are made to feel relaxed and at ease and that the person with whom they talk has a detailed knowledge of aromatherpy. If the patient decides to come for treatment then the consultation procedure will begin.

First, ensure that the treatment room is warm and quiet and gives the atmosphere of peace. The treatment couch needs to be firm and comfortable with suitable drapes. Let the patient undress and lie down, well-covered and warm. Sit beside them and begin quietly to discuss the points outlined below. Having taken name, address and telephone number, and also that of their doctor, then embark on the procedure set out below.

Verbal

One cannot rely entirely on verbal communication, for a variety of reasons. A patient who has come for treatment for the first time might feel shy or even embarrassed and therefore be non-committal in some areas. Also, they may genuinely have forgotten past problems which may have a bearing on their present state of mental and physical health.

There are three areas which need to be approached:

(1) Medical
(2) Social
(3) Family history

The pattern of events leading up to the consultation session will have a profound influence on current wellbeing. Needless to say, problems which have a genuine medical significance must be referred to the General Practitioner before undertaking a treatment programme.

Visual

This is vital for obtaining a correct assessment of the patient's condition. More often than not it is combined with a tactile technique.

Tactile

Tactile adds a third dimension to assessment and a final 'back up' to the information already gained. The areas examined by these last two methods are:

(1) The back
(2) The face
(3) The abdominal area
(4) The feet (reflexology)

The back

The back is the key area for assessment. This is because the nervous system, which controls the whole body, lies within the vertebral column which passes down from the skull to the coccyx. Between each of the vertebrae emerge the spinal nerves which supply action and sensation to all parts of the body. One therefore examines the back as though looking at a map, using it as a guide to explore the functions of all other parts of the body. The methods utilised include checks through visual and tactile techniques on:

(1) Spinal alignment
(2) Colour
(3) Texture
(4) Tension areas of fascia (connective tissue massage)
(5) Pain
(6) 'Flare reaction' by stimulation to circulation

The face

The following points need to be noted:

(1) Colour
(2) Texture
(3) Type
(4) Tone
(5) Expression

The abdominal area

The following points need to be noted:

(1) Pain
(2) Tension

Foot reflexology

The following point needs to be noted:

(1) Reflex pain areas on either foot

Other information

Personality type

The temperament of the patient is taken into account and noted: whether they are 'Yin' (passive, lacking in energy, debilitated) or 'Yang' (active, hypertensive, often irritable and

nervous and certainly prone to stress symptoms). Depending on the personality type, the acupressure techniques are varied, so it is important to know the temperamental characteristics of the patient.

Other information

It is important to know whether the patient is on drugs, medicinal or otherwise, and to find out if there are any other items of medical information which have not been listed.

Precautions – contra indications

It is vital to find out if there are any problem areas before treatment, so that the appropriate oils and massage can be given.

General Practitioner

Should there be a medical problem which should be referred to the doctor before treatment, ensure permission is given in writing.

Full and true facts

Make sure that the patient signs to say that they have given you true and full facts before you give treatment.

Patient responsibility

It is very important to get the patient's signature accepting treatment. Legally this means that they take responsibility for the treatment by aromatherapy.

Oil blends and home care

For each treatment, mark the date of treatment and fill in details of oil blends and homecare advice. Make a note whenever they change according to new patient needs.

Oils

Once all these facts have been correlated, an assessment may be made as to which essential oils and base oils are suitable for the patient's condition. Usually no more than three different oils are required to cope with most of the problems that the therapist can deal with, and these are blended carefully to produce a therapeutic individual blend suitable to that patient alone.

It is important to identify whether it is necessary to have a special facial blend as well as a body blend to ensure that on the consultation accurate formulae are given.

Precautions and contra indications

Aromatherapy massage is an extremely safe treatment when given by a competent, well-trained, qualified aromatherapist. The very small percentage of essential oils in relation to the carrier oil when blended (i.e. $^1/_2$ to 2% maximum of essential oils, namely 3–12 drops maximum in 30 ml of carrier oil) ensures this to be the case.

An aromatherapy massage by a well qualified professional means that there is a 'controlled' use of essential oils. Only 'gross misuse' would cause problems. However, because of the media attention focused on certain oils mentioned in some books on aromatherapy, it is probably sensible for an aromatherapist generally to avoid certain oils for particular conditions, mainly because a perception has been created in the popular mind that there is 'something wrong' with them. This is particularly true of certain oils which some literature claims may have adverse effects in the first three months of pregnancy. Those aromatherapists who have attended courses of a high standard of training will be fully aware of which oils are safe to use for different conditions.

There are certain hazards associated with some oils: toxicity, irritation or sensitisation.

Toxicity

This is commonly called poisoning and at a certain level becomes fatal, whether applied to the skin or taken orally. Toxicity is dose dependent – the greater the amount of essential oil, the greater the hazard. The very small amounts of essential oil put into a carrier oil for an aromatherapy massage by a well-trained professional would not present a problem in any way.

Irritation

There can be localised inflammation affecting the skin or mucous membranes, depending on where the essential oil is applied. Respiratory conditions should be treated with care when using essential oils. The amount of oil(s) chosen, the medium in which it/they are carried and the length of time of inhalation must be safely controlled.

Sensitisation

There can be an allergic response to an essential oil. Only small amounts are required to trigger off a reaction. Photosensitisation occurs when the sun shines on the skin on which certain oils have been applied. A photochemical reaction takes place, causing pigmentation. Bergamot is one of the best known oils which can produce this effect.

Unsafe oils

There are certain oils which present risks either of toxicity, skin irritation or skin sensitisation and are not considered safe in general use.

Not to be used at all in therapy

Almond (bitter)	*Prunus amygdalus var. amara*
Boldo leaf	*Peumus boldus*
Calamus	*Acorus calmus*
Camphor	
brown	*Cinnamomum camphora*
yellow	*Cinnamomum camphora*
Horseradish	*Cochlearia armorica*
Jaborandi leaf	*Pilocarpus jaborandi*
Mugwort (armoise)	*Artemisia vulgaris*
Mustard	*Brassica nigra*
Pennyroyal	
European	*Mentha pulegium*
North American	*Hedeoma pulegioides*
Rue	*Ruta graveolens*
Sassafras	*Sassafras albidum*
Brazilian	*Ocotea cymbarum*
Savin	*Juniperus sabina*
Southernwood	*Artemisia abrotanum*
Tansy	*Tanacetum vulgare*
Thuja	
cedarleaf	*Thuja occidentalis*
plicata	*Thuja plicata*
Wintergreen	*Gaultheria procumbens*
Wormseed	*Chenopodium anthelminticum*
Wormwood	*Artemisia absinthium*

Not to be used on the skin

Cassia	*Cinnamomum cassia*
Clove bud, leaf or stem	*Eugenia caryophyllata*
Cinnamon bark	*Cinnamomum zeylancium*
Costus	*Saussurea lappa*
Elecampane	*Inula helenium*
Fennel (bitter)	*Foeniculam vulgare*
Origanum	*Origanum vulgare*
(Spanish)	*Thymus capitatus*
Pine (dwarf)	*Pinus pumilio*

Savory	
summer	*Satureia hortensis*
winter	*Satureia montana*

Precautions when using essential oils

Apart from these there are certain basic precautions to be taken when using essential oils:

(1) They should not be taken internally unless prescribed by a suitable qualified medical practitioner.

(2) Although the majority of essential oils do not harm the skin, if there is sensitisation or irritation, wash off immediately with mild soap and water.

(3) If an essential oil gets into the eye it may cause pain. Distilled water should be used for washing it out.

(4) Essential oils in most circumstances should be diluted in some carrier medium (vegetable oil, water, cream).

(5) When making up a massage oil the dilution is $1/2$ to 2% (3–12 drops) per 30 ml of carrier oil.

(6) Avoid giving essential oil massage to an acned skin as the passing of the hands may spread infection. Other methods utilising essential oils may be used instead, namely compresses and vaporisers.

(7) Essential oils which are rubifacient in effect should not be used on a dry, sensitive or vaso-dilated skin.

(8) Essential oils should be kept away from flame as they are flammable.

(9) Babies and children need to have a much lower percentage of essential oils to a carrier oil than an adult because of their relatively smaller body area. Usually this would be about 25% of the normal adult dose, and the treatments should be shorter and less frequent.

(10) Medical conditions, if presented on

consultation, should be discussed (with the patient's permission) with their medical practitioner and a written letter of approval received from the medical practitioner before aromatherapy massage is given. In particular, the treatment of a patient with cancer must only be carried out with the approval of the patient's consultant. Some consultants are quite happy to give this approval, others are not, whether the patient is on chemotherapy/radiation therapy or without medication at all. Epilepsy is another state where the oil needs to be selected with care.

As yet there is no complete knowledge of the effects of essential oils combined with massage when a patient is undergoing medical treatment involving drugs. It is imperative therefore that an aromatherapist has the agreement of the patient's medical practitioner before embarking on treatment.

Blending of oils and formulation

When the aromatherapist decides after the consultation with the patient to make up a special blend for that patient's aromatherapy massage, she will know there are two separate components:

(1)   A vegetable carrier oil
(2)   An essential oil or oils incorporated into the carrier oil

Vegetable carrier oil

Many types of carrier oil are available, each useful and having its own properties. These include:

Almond	Softening, soothing to the skin, a light oil suitable for face and body.
Apricot kernel	Deeply penetrating, contains Vitamin A, suitable for the skin and face.
Avocado	Deeply penetrating and very nourishing. Contains Vitamins A and B, is good for dry, mature skin.
Corn	Heavier consistency than almond oil. Nourishing. Best for body treatments.
Grapeseed	Light oil, good for body and face.
Jojoba	Very nourishing oil, which is particularly recommended for dry, mature skins.
Peach kernel	Similar properties to apricot kernel oil.
Safflower	Light and nourishing, recommended for body and face treatments.
Sesame seed	An oil which has the advantage of not staining.
Sunflower	Light and nourishing and good for body and face treatments.
Wheatgerm	Heavy and rather sticky oil. It has Vitamin E which helps to prevent other oil from going rancid. Nourishing to the skin and meant to help with scarring.

Essential oils

Many hundreds are capable of being used, but it is more practical to utilise the better known essential oils.

Formulation

The decision on how to blend the oils depends on the information gained from the patient during the consultation. The important factors are:

(1) The problems discerned during the consultation, which can safely be treated by the aromatherapist

(2) Fragrance appreciation by the patient of the essential oils which the therapist intends to put together in the special blend.

Basic formula

There can be anything from one to five oils in a blend with a carrier oil, but it is usual to have three. This is so that it is possible to cover most problems and at the same time be able to appreciate the subtlety of different essences without finding that they have been swamped. It is usual to put $^1/_2$ to 2% (3 to 12 drops) of essential oils (in total) to an ounce (30 ml) of carrier oil. Fewer drops are required for strong scented oils and more drops for the gentle fragrances.

Each essential oil has many therapeutic values. In making up the special blend it is sensible to write down the problems which you can treat, and against each write a list of the oils which can be helpful in each case. Often it will be seen that a number of oils will be helpful with each of the problems. Provided the fragrances appeal to the patient and blend well together, it is sensible to get maximum benefit by choosing to put these together. Otherwise you can choose an oil suitable for each problem, ensuring that the patient likes each fragrance and that each will blend well with the other(s).

The blend needs to be built up carefully, a drop of each oil at a time. It is wise not to overpower gentle scents such as rose with, for instance, too much eucalyptus. If one wishes to 'fix' the blend it is sensible to incorporate a base note such as patchouli. It is possible to combine any essential oil with any other, but some blend better than others. It takes time and considerable practice to achieve blends which have a harmony of fragrance.

Finally, it is important to remember that the patient's needs may change over successive treatments and that you may have to reformulate the blend accordingly.

Preparation of the patient

After consultation:

(1) The patient lies supine, warm, comfortable and well-covered

(2) A headband is placed on the head to protect hair from creams and oils

(3) The face and neck are deep cleansed with herbal products

(4) The aromatherapy oil is lightly massaged over the face for one minute, with stroking movements

(5) The patient is then asked to move into the prone position, head supported by the hands or a small roll of towelling

Procedure for aromatherapy massage

As stated before, effleurage (stroking) and petrissage (kneading) movements described earlier in this book are techniques often employed by aromatherapists. In addition lymphatic drainage, neuro-muscular and acupressure techniques can be used.

First work on the back, then the backs of the legs, then turn the patient into supine again and commence with the front of the legs, the arms, the abdomen and finish with the scalp, neck, face and shoulders. It must be emphasised that an aromatherapist adapts the massage techniques and the areas treated according to the patient's needs and to any precautions noted in the consultation procedures.

Conclusion

Aromatherapy massage is a safe, useful and effective treatment for a wide variety of conditions, when given by the properly trained therapist. As a result, its role in the health care setting, both in the UK and worldwide, has expanded enormously in the last five years. It is therefore most welcome to see that orthodox and complementary medicine practitioners can work harmoniously together in the further interest of patient care and treatment.

References

Berger, H., Jarosch, E. & Madreiter, W. (1978) Effects of Vapourub and petrolatum on frequency and amplitude of breathing in children with acute bronchitis. *Journal of International Medical Research*, 6, 483–6.

Buchbauer, G., Jirovitz, L., Jager, W. *et al.* (1993) Fragrance compounds and essential oils with sedative effects upon inhalation. *Journal of Pharmacolgical Science*, 82(6), 660–64.

Brun, K. (1952) Les essences vegetales en tant qu'agent de penetration tissulaire. These Pharmacie, Strasbourg.

Cavel, L. (1918) Sur la valeur antiseptique de quelques huiles essentielles. *Comptes Rendus* (Academie des Sciences), 166, 827.

Eysenck, H. (1988) Personality, stress and cancer protection and prophylaxis. *British Journal of Medical and Psychological Science*, 61, 57–75.

Falk-Filipsson, A. (1993) D-limonene exposure to humans by inhalation; uptake, distribution, elimination and effects on the pulmonary system. *Journal of Toxicology and Environmental Health*, 38, 77–88.

Genders, R. (1972) *A History of Scent*, pp. 20 and 126. Hamish Hamilton, London.

Kovar, K.A., Gropper, B., Freiss, D. & Ammon, H.P. (1987) Bloodlevels of 1.8 cineole and locomotor activity of mice, after inhalation and oral administration of rosemary oil. *Planta Medica*, 53(4), 315–18.

Reynolds, P., Boyd, P.T., Blacklow, R.S. *et al.* (1994) The relationship between social ties and survival among black and white breast cancer patients. National Cancer Institute Black/White Cancer Survival Study Group. *Cancer Epidemiology, Biomarkers Prevention*, 3(3), 253–9.

Saller, R., Beschorner, M., Hellenbrecht, D. & Buhrimg, M. (1990) Dose dependency of symptomatic relief of complaints by chamomile steam inhalation in patients with common cold. European Journal of Pharmacology, 183, 728–9.

Schwartz, D. & Natyncuk, S. (eds) (1990) *Chemical Signals in Vertebrates*. Oxford University Press, Oxford.

van Toller, S. & Dodd, G.H. (1988) *Perfumery, the Psychology and Biology of Fragrance*, p. 29. Chapman & Hall, London and New York.

Valnet, Dr Jean (1980) *The Practise of Aromatherapy*, pp. 28, 33, 34. C.W. Daniel, Saffron Walden.

Vickers, A. (1996a) *Massage and Aromatherapy – A Guide for Health Professionals*. Contribution by van Toller, p. 33. Chapman & Hall, London & New York.

Vickers, A. (1996b) *Massage and Aromatherapy – A Guide for Health Professionals*, pp. 174–6. Chapman & Hall, London & New York.

Williams, D. (1989) Lecture Notes on Essential Oils, 19(31), 45. Eve Taylor, London.

Chapter 11
MASSAGE FOR CONDITIONS

Massage for facial palsy

The paralysed muscles of facial expression are treated by using unilateral effleurage, kneading, plucking, reverse hacking and tapping. The normal side of the face should be supported with one hand covered with either a tissue or layer of cotton. Place your little finger on the chin, your ring finger on the upper lip and your middle and index fingers on the cheek with your thumb on the forehead. Apply a slight downwards and medial pressure towards mid-line of the face, and maintain it while giving the massage to the paralysed side.

Additional manipulation – eye closing

Place one forefinger along the upper eyelid and gently close and open it several times. This manoeuvre helps to lubricate the eyeball. Teach the patient to perform this manipulation.

Massage using lubricants

Preparation

Of the patient

Support the area to be treated, and ensure his or her general comfort. Spread under the area a protective, waterproof sheeting covered with either a washable sheet or towel, or a disposable sheet. Uncover the area.

Of the tray

This should be suitably adjacent to the area to be treated.

using lanolin
 – the lanolin or lanolin cream
 – a bowl of swabs
 – a receiver for dirty swabs

using oil
 – the oil
 – small dish or container
 – bowl of swabs
 – receiver for dirty swabs

using soap and oil
 – the oil
 – small dish or container
 – bowl of swabs
 – dish containing non-caustic soap
 – bowl of hand-hot water (the hottest your palm will tolerate)
 – receptable for dirty swabs
 – hand towel

Of the practitioner

Remove rings and wristwatch, and ensure your nails are short. Try to sit down so that you can relax and maintain a prolonged treatment without undue fatigue.

The treatment

Using oil or lanolin or ung. eucerin

Open the container and leave the cap off. If using oil, pour a little into the dish.

Examine the part to be treated and using your finger or thumb tips apply the lubricant to the margins, then to the centre of the area. If possible, support your forearms or elbows adjacent to the treatment area and, using your lubricated finger or thumb tips, work from the periphery to the centre of the area.

As you work, the lubricant may 'disappear' so add more, a small amount at a time, on the area on which you are at present working. Do not at any point swamp or flood the area.

On completion:

either leave the residual lubricant on the skin
or gently swab most of it away, using a clean swab for each subsection cleaned, and wiping the central area first followed by the margins.

Using soap and oil

Open the container of oil and pour a little into the small dish. Put the **palmar surface only** of your hands on to the surface of the hot water, so that the dorsal surface does not become wet. Use the soap to work up a good lather on the front of your hands. Pour about 5 ml (one teaspoon) of oil on to the palm of one hand, and work your palms together to distribute the oil into the lather.

Apply your hands to the area to be treated, spreading the lather over the whole area. If you need more lather repeat the above procedure, but you will find the lather spreads over a large area. Now, work with one or both hands over the whole area using stroking or kneading type manipulations. The object is not to work deeply, but to spread the lather and loosen scales of skin. As the scaly patches are loosened, use a swab to remove them from the work area.

If the lather dries up or disappears, remoisten your palms and work them together first. You may find the lather reforms, but if not recreate lather by following the above procedure.

On completion of the treatment:

either wipe the whole area with swabs, working on a whole limb from proximal to distal, or on a smaller part from centre to periphery. This will leave a thin coat of oil on the area.
or wash the area by first washing your own hands and rinsing them, then lathering them so that you can apply a non-oily lather to the part to wash it.

Rinse, swab clean as above, then dry the part if necessary.

Massage for scars, burns and plastic surgery

All scars, whether primary lesions, secondary repairs or grafts, have a tendency to contract by as much as a third of their length. All injuries to the skin, whatever the cause, also tend to become oedematous, and may become slow-healing and indurated. The oedema can be a disaster in the case of a skin graft which may be 'lifted' and prevented from 'taking' by the oedema.

At best, permanently contracted scars will cause inconvenience and at worst they cause gross deformities with severe functional limitation.

Along with other measures, the appropriate application of suitable massage techniques will help to maintain scar length and assist the movement of oedema so that it may be resolved or absorbed. The appropriate moment at which to massage any scar, healing burn or plastic repair will be determined by the state of the healing process, the other underlying injuries or lesions and the imperative need to prevent the above complications. It must be borne in mind that over-zealous and too early massage may encourage the formation of hypertrophic (keloid) tissue to which burns victims are especially prone.

Contact materials are usually used as they lubricate the skin, allow gliding without friction and often make painful manipulations more tolerable. The different oils and their uses are explained on p. 144, and it should be noted that where wounds are still unhealed, great care must be taken to avoid infection. The selected lubricant should be sterile and renewed daily or at each treatment, and it should be used only up to the margin and not over the open wound.

The massage manipulations which are used are those suitable to treat the state at that moment. Thus, the initial or persistent oedema must be treated by clearing the venous and lymphatic vessels proximal to the wound, using the techniques described for oedema on p. 148. The localised area of oedema may need fingertip vibrations, effleurage strokes initially at the margins and gradually encroaching on to the more central area, followed by finger or thumb kneading interspersed with effleurage strokes, until the swelling is softer and the patient tolerates handling better.

Next, use as much of your hand as possible to apply pressure over a larger area (Fig. 11.1). The central (unhealed) area may be covered with a sterile dressing and gently kneaded, maintaining even pressure and attempting to compress and move the whole scarred and swollen area. Rocking the whole area may be feasible, using your hands as in muscle rolling (Fig. 2.25). Complete your work, by effleurage strokes from distal, round the scar to the prox-

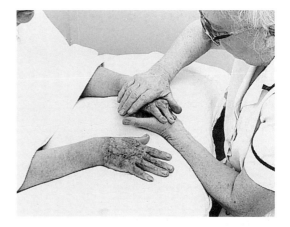

Fig. 11.1 Compressive palmar kneading to the dorsum of a burnt and grafted hand.

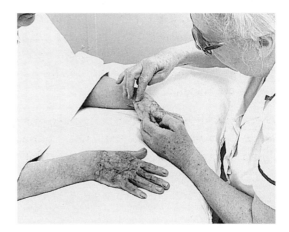

Fig. 11.2 Finger kneading to the periphery of the burnt hand.

imal lymph glands, including the scar in the strokes if possible. It may be necessary to work more lightly over the scar itself with these strokes.

The scar which is less oedematous but more bound down or contracted greatly, is treated by initial and gradually deepening effleurage strokes round the periphery, followed by finger and thumb tip kneading to the same area (Figs 11.2, 11.3, 11.4). Then, work on to the scar with the small kneading manipulations, continuing

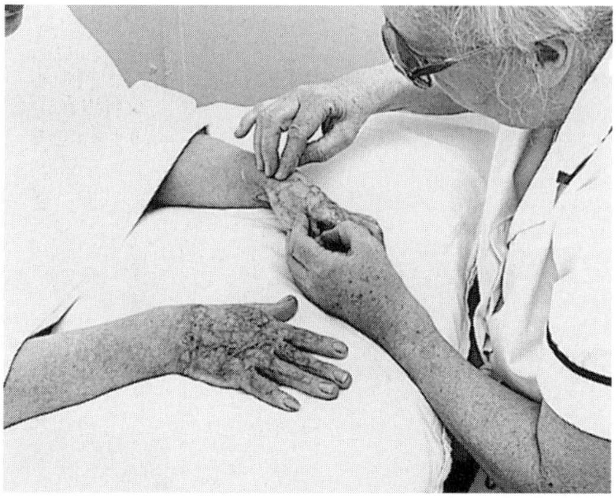

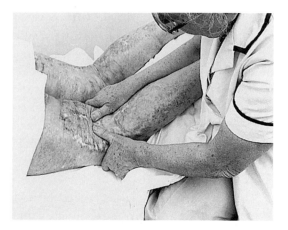

Fig. 11.3 Encroaching and deepening the finger kneading.

Fig. 11.5 Stroking the central area. Note that the wrinkle at the thumb tips indicates some skin mobility.

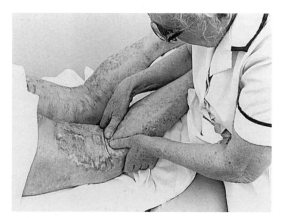

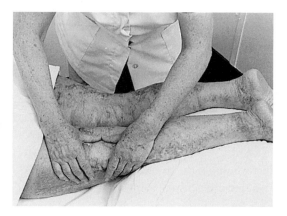

Fig. 11.4 Thumb kneading to the central and more mobile area of burns to the back of the knee.

Fig. 11.6 Rocking the whole area from side to side.

until the skin is either warmer to touch or pink, or both. Start slowly and increase your speed as the patient's tolerance increases.

Now start to use stretching manipulations, which may be finger or thumb tip kneading with greater depth and slightly greater range, or stretching strokes (Fig. 11.5), working along the length of the scar and gradually using the side of your thumb or finger to push up against the scar as you stroke along the margin.

Intersperse with rocking the whole scar (Fig. 11.6) along its length from side to side using either one or both hands, and then attempt small wringing manipulations (Figs 11.7 and 11.8). Identify the worst areas and give them special attention, perform local skin wringing and skin rocking, and finish with effleurage round and to the whole area from distal to it, and up to the proximal lymph glands.

In some cases, you may find it better to

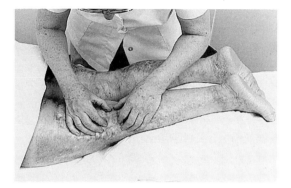

Fig. 11.7 Wringing a small area using finger and thumb tips on the back of the knee.

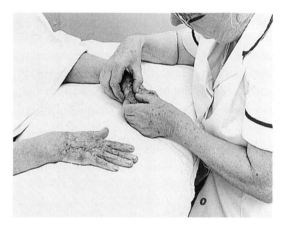

Fig. 11.8 Wringing on the side of the hand to mobilise the adherent skin.

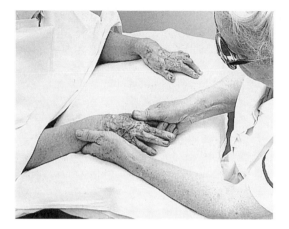

Fig. 11.9 Squeeze kneading to each finger with stretch on the tip to maintain extension.

At the completion of the massage, the surplus lubricant may be wiped off with the swabs, or may be left on the skin to facilitate its lubrication. The patient should, if possible, be taught to use a selection of appropriate manipulations on his or her own scars.

Treatment for haematoma

Painful areas may be treated by massage in an attempt to relieve the pain. Areas of disorder often have local spasm which is protective. As the attempt to protect against movement of the part spreads, yet more spasm will spread to the adjacent areas. Spasm prevents drainage and thus causes local congestion. Metabolites accumulate and increase the disorder and discomfort.

Bruising or haematoma are the consequence of injury and may both present at the site of the injury, and in adjacent or distal areas into which the extravasated blood will spread. It is important to differentiate between the local haematoma at the site of the injury, which should not be treated for up to four days until damaged small blood vessels have had time to

support the more distal part of a limb manually and apply stretch with your supporting hand as the tissues become warm and softer (Figs 11.8 and 11.9). The stretch should be so gentle as to be unobtrusive and should not make the patient aware of increased discomfort.

In the section on kneading in Chapter 2, it was stressed that the circling of the hand should avoid sudden points and becoming pear shaped. In working to stretch scars by kneading, a more pear shaped manipulation should be cultivated, the 'point' of the pear shape being the moment of greatest stretch on the tissues.

heal, and the more distant accumulation of extravasated blood, which may show as swelling as well as bruising. This oedema may be treated early to avoid consolidation, but care must be taken to cause no drag or pull on the site of the lesion. The techniques described below should be used.

The local bruised area which may well be painful, and the painful areas described in the first paragraph, can be treated in a similar manner.

Start proximal to the lesion and clear the proximal structures using effleurage, kneading and possibly picking up. Then work round the affected area, initially not touching it, but using stationary finger, thumb or palmar kneading, followed by small strokes of effleurage with the same hand component from the area worked upon to a more proximal normal area. If the patient will tolerate it, gradually encroach on the margins and then the more central part of the affected area using the same techniques. If, however, the area is very tense and painful, place as much of your hand as possible over the area and give vibrations. Keep on with the vibrations until you feel the area becoming less tense, when it may be possible to use gentle finger or thumb kneadings to the margins and work inwards.

Another useful local manipulation is gentle rocking of the area. This is especially helpful on a bruise or local swelling. Place your hand so as to encompass the whole area and gently move the mass sideways. Initially the rocking must be gentle and not too deep, but eventually depth can be increased and your hand can move up and down the area as in rocking, described on p. 146.

Intersperse the rocking with short strokes of effleurage and more kneading on the margins of the affected area, continuing until you feel softening of the tissues, diminution of tension and the patient experiences relief of pain. Persistent

thickenings may be treated by using circular frictions with great care. Again, start around the margin and encroach to the centre and intersperse with effleurage strokes towards the nearest lymph glands.

Massage for oedema

There are two extremes of oedema: that which is softer, mobile and usually of recent origin, and that which is consolidated, indurated and usually of much longer standing. Oedema may present at any stage between these states. The earlier it can be treated, the better the result is likely to be (Boyce 1996).

Any restrictive clothing should be removed from the area proximal to the oedema so that drainage is facilitated. All oedematous areas should be elevated for a time (usually one hour) prior to massage.

The elevation should be such that the limb is supported at an angle of about 45° to the horizontal, and care must be taken that the trunk and head are not also raised causing an increase in this angle. Thus, the patient should lie as flat as possible, using pillows to support the head and not to elevate the trunk. Each part of the limb under treatment should be elevated more than the next most proximal part, to allow drainage through the increasingly large veins and lymph vessels and through the lymph glands (Fig. 5.1).

The patient should be encouraged to help during elevation, massage and afterwards, by performing a series of deep breathing exercises. The effect of a deep breath is to cause a lowering of the negative pressure in the mediasteinum, so that lymph and venous blood at a higher pressure in adjacent areas will flow to the lower pressure area.

Some massage manipulations can be combined with active contraction of the muscles under treatment, and at the end of the massage regime active exercises should be taught with stress on slow, sustained contractions and relaxation, and regular repetition throughout the day.

Pressure garments should be applied before the patient moves.

The area proximal to the oedematous area should be treated by all manipulations that will assist drainage, to leave clear passage for the accumulated fluids. The drainage should be facilitated by clearing the lymph sheds of the trunk (Casley-Smith 1994), initially the area furthest from the oedematous area and draining into the opposite lymph glands. Remember that although lymphatics have valves normally controlling one-way flow, during engorgement the glands are ineffective and flow can be in any direction and will respond to a pumping type of pressure.

Thus for a swollen left arm, the right upper trunk is treated first (Gillam 1994) followed by the left upper trunk, with the flow directed horizontally to the right axilla. The left upper arm is then treated sectionally (Fig. 11.10). For the lower limb, the area of trunk below the axilla on the opposite side, then the same side, is cleared first, followed by progressively distal areas of the trunk before the lower limb is treated (Fig. 11.11).

The manipulations should be to both the lymph vessels and the nodes which require localised stationary kneading. The whole treatment must be gentle so as to avoid further damage, especially when the oedema is recent and/or soft. The manipulations used are a firm unidirectional stroke gradually becoming deeper on the trunk. Each stroke should overlap the previous one and the stationary fingertip kneading to the lymph glands should be interspersed with the stroking.

Effleurage, slow deep kneading with extra compression, and slow compressive picking up should be performed from the most proximal lymph glands (groin or axilla) to the part where the oedema starts. Each effleurage stroke should be accompanied by a deep inspiration, both timed for maximum inspiration by the time of arrival of your hands at the appropriate group of lymph glands (space).

The treatment of the oedematous area will differ with the type of oedema but the basic rules are the same for any type of oedema. The area is treated one hand width at a time. Each hand width is constantly drained as the oedema is softened and moved so that it is included in effleurage strokes to the most proximal area.

The more proximal oedematous area should be regarded as having four aspects like a four-sided tube, and opposing aspects are handled together. Thus, aspect **one** is treated with counterpressure on opposite area **three**. Then area **three** is treated with counterpressure on area **one**. The same manipulation is performed on areas **two** and **four**, before the manipulation is changed for a deeper or more mobilising technique. All manipulations in which the tissues are moved sideways are initially performed very slowly.

The manipulations which are of use on **soft** oedema are:

(1) Vibrations performed single-handed with opposite counterpressure on each aspect, followed by double-handed vibrations on opposite aspects.

(2) As the tissues become less tense, a very small range, stationary, single handed kneading can be performed, first on one aspect then the opposite, then on the two sides together. Intersperse this manipulation with effleurage, and increase the size of the hand circling, as the tissue mobility increases.

(3) If the oedema is in the deeper tissues, a squeeze kneading may be used. Place your

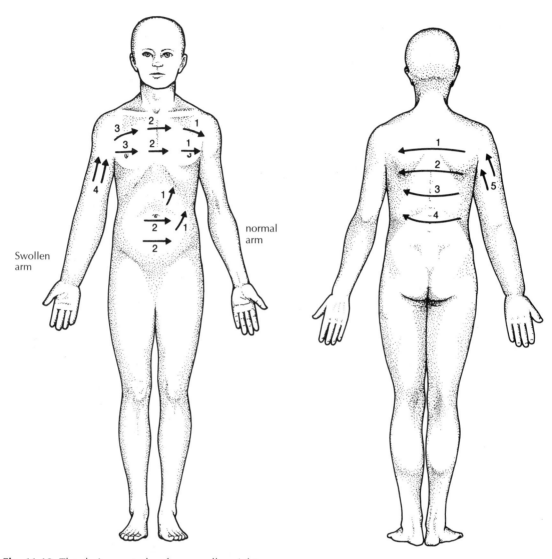

Fig. 11.10 The drainage strokes for a swollen right arm.

two hands on opposite aspects of the part in firm and complete contact, with your index fingers more proximal. Now exert more pressure successively with your hand in the line of the little, ring, middle and index fingers, i.e. the finger and area of palm proximal to it press together. The pressure is maintained with each component as the squeeze extends until the whole hand is exerting pressure. Thus,

any fluid is squeezed onwards by the width of your hand. Effleurage again.

(4) Still working in a box formation, stationary double-handed kneading can be performed on all four aspects, with an increasing depth and range of manipulation.

(5) Then, move on to the next hand width down the part and repeat the manipulations, working gradually over the oedematous area.

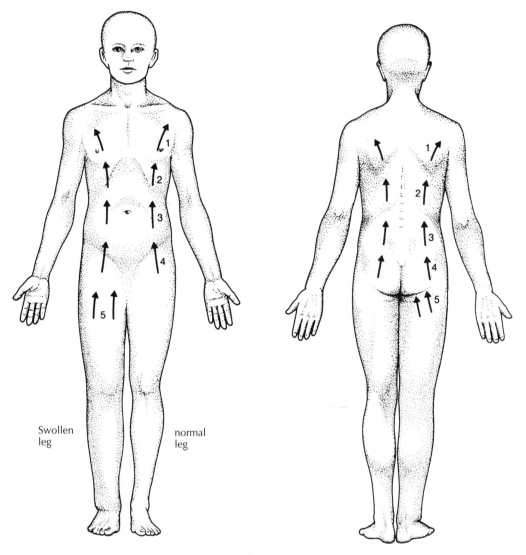

Fig. 11.11 The drainage strokes for a swollen right leg.

The ankle and foot

In spite of oedema which rounds the contours, this area presents special problems as only the sole of the foot is muscular, and the shape of the parts requires special disposition of the hands.

The same manipulations are used, in the same manner and order, but one of your hands may well encompass the front and sides of the ankle, while the other treats the medial and lateral aspects of the tendocalcaneal area (often called the medial and lateral coulisse), using the length of your thumb and thenar eminence on one side, and on the other two distal phalanges of all four fingers, flexed at the proximal interphalangeal joints. In effect, a triangular plan of action should be evolved, and you should additionally use your flat fingers or palms according to the way they fit on the area under treatment.

On the foot, the sole is given constant counterpressure, as, if the patient is ambulant, the compressive force of weightbearing will stop oedema accumulating under the foot. Treatment is then directed at the dorsum of the foot and at the toes.

The wrist and hand

The more confined area of the wrist and hand, even when swollen, will require disposition of your hands in opposite directions so as to encompass the area. One hand is placed vertically on one aspect, and the other hand is wrapped horizontally round the opposite side of the limb. This hand disposition can be used for the same sequence of manipulations as on the proximal areas. Unlike the sole of the foot, the palm of the hand can become swollen and require treatment. The digits are each long enough to be squeezed using one hand on each digit, and the dorsum of the hand is usually treated initially using your palm, and eventually the length of the sides of your thumbs in the interosseus spaces.

As each area is treated, encourage active movements of the joints of that part. If necessary, demonstrate the required movement passively a few times, then require slow, active movements with a 'holding' (isometric) contraction at the end of the range in each direction. These contractions can be enhanced by a firm squeeze knead performed at the same time.

The manipulations which are of use on **consolidated** oedema are:

(1)   Single-handed kneading with as large a range as the tissue state allows; opposite compression is essential
(2)   Alternate double-handed kneading on opposite aspects followed by simultaneous double-handed kneading
(3)   If any softening of tissues occur, squeeze

kneading may be performed and interspersed with effleurage

Eventually, kneading may be increased in depth and range until the tissues feel softer.

Massage for relaxation

All massage manipulations used to induce relaxation should be performed to two rules:

(1)   The tempo should be slow
(2)   The repetition of each manipulation should continue without interruption or change until either the practitioner detects a reduction in tension, or feels the palmar surface of his or her hands becoming numbed. Thus, the patient might be equally aware of numbness.

In addition, your own movements should be smooth and rhythmical. Local relaxation techniques may be applied to any part of the body, obeying the basic rules of making the model/patient comfortable and adopting a position yourself in which you can sustain a prolonged performance of the chosen manipulation. For most areas, the manipulations to be performed would be in one of these orders:

either:	*or*:
• Stroking	• Effleurage
• Kneading	• Kneading
• Effleurage	

The choice will depend partly on the recipient's response to stroking – some people dislike being stroked from proximal to distal – when effleurage would be substituted; and partly on the reasons for using a relaxation massage. It may be that a painful, congested area will not relax until it is decongested, when effleurage may be used first. In some cases it may even be necessary to start with stationary vibrations, followed by labile vibrations when a stroke is made as the vibrations are performed. This manipulation is excellent when the skin is very tender to touch, in addition to the painful underlying spasm.

Stroking and effleurage must be performed with great smoothness and no flourish of the hands at the beginning or end of each line of work. Kneading must be at sufficient depth not to tickle, and must be very even throughout the length of the line of work. Your hand movements between manipulations must be calm and unhurried and within the tempo of the work being performed. It is sometimes advisable to tell the patient when a change of work is to be effected, but this should not be done when attempting to obtain general relaxation by treating either the whole neck and back, or by whole body stroking.

Whole body relaxation can sometimes be gained by performing a sedative massage to the back and neck, more especially so if the patient can be made comfortable in the prone lying position. Some patients find impossible the use of an active technique of relaxation by some form of muscle action and relaxation, or by posture or by meditative methods, and they may respond to whole body stroking. Ask the patient to remove some outer clothing, and to lie down either prone or in side lying. Cover him or her from neck to toes with a blanket, and tuck it in firmly over the neck. Take up a long, lunge standing position at the side of the plinth near the lower limbs (Fig. 1.1), and check that you can reach forwards to the shoulder and turn your hands and body to reach the feet (avoid the soles). Now work out a pattern so that you stroke over every part of the body equally, e.g.:

patient in prone lying
 – one hand each side of centre back
 – one hand each side over scapulae
 – one hand each side in line with axillae
 – one hand each side down arms and outer sides of legs

patient in lying
 – follow a similar pattern (use a curved line of work outwards or inwards round the breasts)

patient in side lying
 – either work single-handed on the back or single-handed on the front, or one hand each side covering opposite areas.

These patterns mean both hands work together, and you must exert good control over both your movements, posture and the downward pull you exert to keep the movement smooth and of even depth. The human body can have quite sharp hillocks and valleys when lying down for this treatment, and it is easy to do fast downhill runs and bump at the valley bottom.

Some patients prefer a single-handed pattern of work – one stroke to the right and one to the left. This technique may be forced on a small practitioner treating a tall patient, when you will increase your reach by rotating your trunk as well as reaching with your upper limb.

A technique called 'thousand hands' is sometimes used to overcome reaching problems. Each hand in turn performs a short stroke, each stroke overlapping that previously performed by two-thirds of its length.

Total relaxation may be induced in some very tense patients by giving them a very slow facial massage, or by a sedative massage to the neck with the patient in lying as in Fig. 6.1. When using this position it is easily feasible to work on the suboccipital muscles, especially those forming the suboccipital triangle, and the position and technique is helpful for posterior tension headaches.

Using the percussive manipulations on the thorax

(Practise this first on a model.)

Percussive manipulations and vibrations are used to assist patients to evacuate secretions.

Any of the percussive manipulations may be used to help to remove secretions and they should usually be performed over a thin covering to reduce skin effects. They are frequently combined with postural drainage so the patient should first be placed in the pre-determined drainage position, which should if possible allow you to see the patient's face. Cover the area to be treated with a thin blanket or single layer of sheet or towel and ensure it is smooth (Fig. 2.34). Warn the patient the treatment is likely to be noisy and will be deep. Try to stand in such a position that the patient cannot breathe on you.

Clapping is performed by placing one or both hands in position and initiating the deeper clap described on pp. 25–26 (Figs 2.33 and 2.34). Clap more lightly than your planned eventual depth. Gradually work more deeply and try to intersperse your work with encouragement to the patient to cough by using long, expiratory breaths or by huffing.

Over the smaller areas, such as the apices of the lungs, single-handed work may be all that is possible. Double-handed work is feasible over the area of the lower lobes of the lungs, and your hands may be able to move forwards and backwards on the lower rib cage. The depth effect you should try to obtain is that of slight jarring of the chest. It is sometimes likened to the sharp blows struck on the bottom of a newly started or nearly empty sauce bottle. Think of trying to jerk sticky secretions off the lung tissue to which they are adhering, and aim for a loosening effect.

Hacking is performed in similar areas, but allows both hands to be used in smaller areas such as over the lung apices. The depth effect is much less, but may be sufficiently effective on the very young patient, or safer on those who have a tendency to osteoporotic bones (Fig. 2.36).

Beating and/or pounding are alternatives which give your hands a rest. Beating may also give you very localised greater depth and can be used to dislodge obstructive secretions or inhaled objects. Pounding is certainly less tiring on your fingertips than hacking, and can be used on smaller areas as a variation from hacking, and to obtain more depth. The mode of performance is described and illustrated in Chapter 2, Figs 2.38 and 2.39.

Chest vibrations

As with the percussive manipulations, the patient is placed in a predetermined position which either enables him or her to cough more effectively, or allows gravity to assist the drainage of secretions.

One side of the chest is usually treated at a time. If the patient is very small, for example a baby, you will find the whole chest can be completely covered by your hand, but you must in such cases avoid treating both lungs at once by using only part of your hand. The smaller the chest, the more important it is that you give only vibrations and do not exert a squeeze which obstructs respiration and can cause a great increase in the heart rate.

For the apex of one lung

Place your hands, one at the front and one at the back, over the area of the lung apex. Your anterior hand should have the fingertips resting below the clavicle, and you must avoid compression of breast tissue. To this end, keep your hand oblique so that your palm is more lateral than your fingers. Your posterior hand should be at a higher level as in Fig. 11.12.

For the middle lobes of the lung (left lingula)

Place your hands, one at the front and one at the back, as in Fig. 11.13, so that your rear hand lies over the area occupied by the lower half of the scapula. If necessary, the patient's scapula can be protracted by stretching his or her arm forwards, to allow your rear hand to lie over some part of ribs 3–7. Your front hand should cover the same ribs in such a manner as to avoid the breast. Your two thumbs should be adjacent to each other in the mid-axillary line.

For the lower lobes of the lung

With your thumbs adjacent in the mid-axillary line, place your hands along the line of ribs 6–10. Your front hand should be below the breast and along the line of the costal cartilages, while your rear hand should be along the line of the ribs (Fig. 11.14).

The vibrations are first given without commanded respiratory action, but will be more effective if each burst of vibration is in time with the patient's expiration and if the burst of vibration lasts for the whole expiratory phase. You should rest on each inspiratory phase.

Initially, vibrate gently first with one hand, then the other, then both together. The single-handed work allows you to explore the patient's relaxation and rigidity of the chest wall. It also accustoms the patient to your touch and to the manipulation. As you start the double-handed work, ensure that you maintain an even pressure with all parts of your hand which are in contact. Be especially careful to avoid excess pressure with the heels of your hands. Under no circumstances should your hands shake sideways, which will be ineffective.

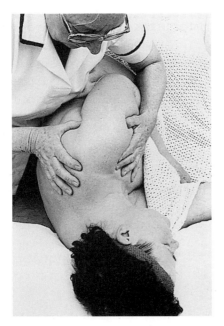

Fig. 11.12 Chest vibrations – hand positions for the apex of the lungs.

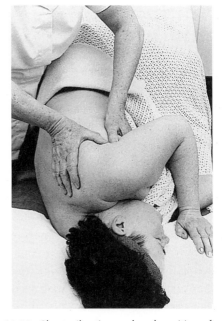

Fig. 11.13 Chest vibrations – hand positions for the middle areas of the lungs.

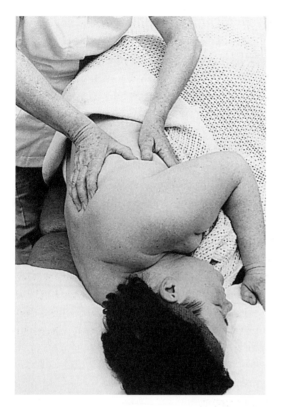

Fig. 11.14 Chest vibrations – hand positions for the basal areas of the lungs.

The vibratory action must be in and out with your hands, so that you obtain a fast vibratory action of your hands towards one another, and through the patient's chest. Try to increase your depth a little as the expiration proceeds. A greater increase in depth is possible when the patient can perform active expirations as you perform the vibrations and follow the inward movement of the chest wall. At the end of the expirations, hold the compressive pressure of your hands (**do not jerk**) for a short interval, and then release your hand pressure suddenly. The patient will breathe in. If the patient wishes to cough, you can assist by holding your pressure without vibrations. It is also most important to avoid exerting pressure which is more inclined to push the whole

thorax into the bed, instead of giving pressure only through the chest wall.

The amount of inward movement of the chest wall which you can obtain will be greatest at the lung bases, and will be less at the lung apices. The range of movement will also be less in the elderly, and in those with chronic chest conditions.

Connective tissue massage

Connective tissue massage is a very specialised technique, first used on herself by Elizabeth Dicke of Germany. The work done by the Germans resulted in the method known as connective tissue massage, fully described by the late Maria Ebner FCSP (Holey 1995). Briefly, the technique aims at mobilising the deep, reticular layer of the dermis where the gel-like, ground substance is found, and is strongly related to the multiple links between the autonomic and somatic systems.

This system is dependent on thorough examination of the patient in sitting as in Fig. 11.15, starting with inspection of the back to identify alterations in contour due to flattening or elevation caused by the changes in other structures supplied by that dermatome.

Manual examination follows, to investigate the mobility of the various layers of connective tissue, and the tension present in the muscular layers. A pattern of examination is followed which includes lifting and stroking manipulations along the paravertebral area.

The manual technique used for treatment is performed with the middle finger, using either the tip or the finger pad extending the length of the distal phalanx on the radial side. Moderate touch is applied to the patient's skin to obtain adherence (never use lubricants), and the middle finger is supported by the distal phalanx of the ring finger. The fingertip is applied at an

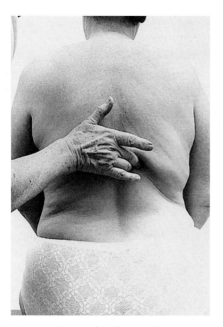

Fig. 11.15 Position and technique for connective tissue massage.

- Varying the speed of the stroke
- Shortening the stroke
- Varying the depth by altering the angle of the hand (decrease in the angle decreases the depth, and increase in the angle increases the depth).

The strokes are performed in the lines of the dermatomes, towards the mid-line in the paravertebral areas and in the direction of the muscle fibres in peripheral areas.

On the back, the right side is treated with the practitioner's right hand and the left side with the practitioner's left hand. On the periphery, the appropriate hand to the practitioner's position in relation to the patient is used. Ebner stresses that the appropriate paravertebral dermatomes should always be treated before the peripheral work is undertaken.

angle of 45° to the skin (Fig. 11.15), and the slack is taken out of the superficial tissue. A pull is exerted in the direction of the desired stroke, with the radial or anterior side of the wrist joint leading, so that the superficial connective tissue is moved on the deeper connective tissue. A ripple of skin should move before the stroking finger. The patient should feel only a sensation of touch, or a slight scratching or cutting sensation. More severe sensations may indicate a need for revision of technique by:

References

Boyce, G. (1996) Lymphoedema – Palliative Physiotherapy. *Medicine Australia*.

Casley-Smith, J.R. (1994) *Modern Treatment for Lymphoedema*. Research paper, the Henry Thomas Laboratory of Australia, pp. 117, 130, 225.

Gillam, L. (1994) Lymphoedema and physiotherapists, control not cure. *Physiotherapy*, 8(12).

Holey, L. (1995) *Connective Tissue Massage*. R.G. Krieger Publishing Company, Mababar, Florida.

INDEX